HEALING AS A PARISH MINISTRY

LEO THOMAS, O.P.
and JAN ALKIRE

HEALING AS A PARISH MINISTRY

Mending Body, Mind, and Spirit

Byron Books   Seattle, WA 98115-1072

Excerpts from *Peace, Love, and Healing* by Bernie S. Siegel,
© copyright 1989, Harper and Row, New York. Used with permission.

Unless otherwise noted, all excerpts are from THE NEW JERUSALEM
BIBLE, copyright © 1985 by Darton, Longman & Todd, Ltd. and Doubleday
& Company, Inc. Reprinted by permission of the publisher.

IMPRIMI POTEST:
    The Very Reverend Daniel Syverstad, O.P.
    Prior Provincial
    Province of the Most Holy Name of Jesus, Oakland, CA
    December 4, 1999

NIHIL OBSTAT:
    Fabian Parmisano, O.P.
    Censor deputatus

Byron Books   Box 51072
                  Seattle, WA 98115-1072

International Standard Book Number: 0-9679815-0-6
(first published in 1991 by Ave Maria Press, ISBN 0-87793-474-6)

Library of Congress Catalog Card Number: 00-102891

Cover design by Marci Mill

Cover photograph by Fred Alkire

Printed and bound in the United States of America by QMedia, Inc.

We dedicate this book to all the people in the Institute for Christian Ministries — staff members, students, and graduates.

> We always thank God for you all, mentioning you in our prayers continually. We remember before our God and Father how active is the faith, how unsparing the love, how persevering the hope which you have from our Lord Jesus Christ (1 Thes 1:2–3).

ABOUT THE AUTHORS

Leo Thomas, O.P. (1922-1997) wrote *Healing Ministry: A Practical Guide* (Sheed & Ward, 1994), co-authored "Formation for Healing Ministry" (see below), and founded the Institute for Christian Ministries. Father Thomas spent over 35 years in the ministry of pastoral care.

Jan Alkire is a freelance writer, a former physical therapist, a teacher with the Institute for Christian Ministries, and co-author of "Formation for Healing Ministry".

ABOUT THE INSTITUTE FOR CHRISTIAN MINISTRIES

The Institute for Christian Ministries (ICM) was founded in 1977 by Father Thomas to help Christians minister together so that hurting people can experience the healing love of God. Teaching from a Roman Catholic perspective while valuing and respecting all Christian traditions, ICM has trained over 2,000 people from many Christian faiths. For more about ICM and its program, please see its website: **http://www.healingministry.org**

RESOURCES FOR FURTHER GROWTH BY THE AUTHORS

Healing Ministry: A Practical Guide (Sheed & Ward, 1994). A pastoral care resource for individuals and groups. Topics include: ministering as a team, listening in ways that promote healing, different kinds of wounds and remedies, and a chapter on spiritual gifts. Also included: reflection questions at the end of each chapter.

Formation for Healing Ministry (Institute for Christian Ministries, 1997 and 1998). FHM is an in-depth, parish-based program whose goal is spiritual formation in preparation for being competent ministers of religious healing. FHM is the published version of a program taught for 23 years in the Pacific Northwest by Father Thomas. It now is available to Christian communities in their own geographic area. For further information or to acquire the program, please see ICM's website: **http://www.healingministry.org**

Contents

Introduction

We have written this book to give caring Christians a pastorally sound guide that draws upon the richness of our communal Christian heritage. The writing process itself showed us the added power of serving God in union with other believers, because both of us made specific contributions in collaborating on this project.

Leo contributed his teaching gifts as a Dominican priest, plus his experience (since 1954) in pastoral care. Five years of this time was spent on the staff of the Department of Pastoral Care at the Menninger Foundation. Another five years was spent developing and directing a pastoral training program for Dominican priests. The knowledge gained from training priests in pastoral care led Leo to launch a similar program for laity. In conjunction with several dedicated lay people, in 1978 he founded the Institute for Christian Ministries (ICM), a two-year program which trains Christians for religious healing ministry.

Jan's major contribution to this book was her professional writing skill. In addition, she brought her experiences as a physical therapist, wife, mother, active parishioner, ICM teacher, and prayer minister. The many narratives found within these chapters sprang from both of our encounters with life in general, and with ministers and hurting people in particular.

The collaboration process evolved into a sentence-by-sentence consensus. Leo's background and insights merged with Jan's writing and life experiences to produce the "third voice" that co-authors often discover.

To preserve confidentiality, we have taken considerable pains to disguise the stories we have used in this book. Except in these few instances where we had the party's consent to use the material, all stories are composites of typical cases, representing no one person. If you think you recognize yourself or another person in an anecdote, it is only because of the commonality of human experiences that we all share. We have used fictitious names except for ourselves and our colleagues in the Institute for Christian Ministries.

A Word About Words

The English language has a problem: no pronoun exists that expresses both male *and* female. Therefore any pronoun that writers apply to the divine will always fall short because God transcends gender but contains the depths of both the masculine and the feminine.

Some writers cope with this problem by avoiding all pronouns that refer to the Lord. Instead, they use the noun "God." As a result, "God" can appear in a sentence five or six times, until it is modifying itself and giving the impression that more than one God exists! (e.g., "God reveals God's will to us.) In the laudable quest for inclusive language, prose can suffer. We wrestled with this no-win situation and decided that when necessary, we would use traditional pronouns to refer to God.

Writers face another version of the male-and-female pronoun deficit when they hunt for one that expresses male *or* female. Our solution for this book was to alternate between masculine and feminine pronouns when referring to a non-specific person.

As co-authors, we use "we" to indicate both of us, "Leo" to specify only Leo, and "Jan" to denote only Jan.

Finally, in this book "minister" means any ministering person without reference to ordination, and "supplicant" means the recipient of ministry.

Chapter One

Healing in the Parish

What healing ministry is taking place in today's parishes, and how can this grow?

The stooped, silver-haired parishioner arrived at the priory asking for a key. While Leo hunted it down, Jan listened to the man's rapid-fire commentary about anything and everything in life. Suddenly he stopped, stared at Jan and said, "Say, why are *you* here, anyway?" "A priest and I are working on a book about healing," she said. "Oh, you mean 'charismatic' healing?" he responded, struggling with the word charismatic. "Religious healing," replied Jan. "Jesus did a lot of it when he was on earth." The man crossed his arms, squinted up at the ceiling for a moment, then finally said, "Healing. I don't know what to say about healing."

He's not alone. Although religious healing is a 2,000-year-old treasure in the Catholic church, it has been pastorally ignored for several centuries. Outside of charismatic circles, few people know what to say about it. When they do speak, they tend to label it a "marginal issue," right over there next to forecasting the end of the world.

The absence of healing ministry at the parish level deprives people of access to the healing power of Christ. Jesus commissioned his disciples to "cure the sick, raise the dead, cleanse the lepers, cast out devils" (Mt 10:8a, *JB*). Most of today's parishioners lack an experience of God meeting these needs in their lives. They rarely say this directly, but if we examine our parishes carefully, the evidence surrounds us. We can see scenarios such as these:

• A woman named Dorothy comes to mass each Sunday, but she never receives communion. She sits at the back of the church, avoids eye contact or conversation with anyone, and sometimes weeps. Obviously she is deeply distressed and alienated. How can the faith community help her?

• Once a year, St. Mary's administers the sacrament of anointing of the sick after its 10:00 mass. Father Jim gives a homily during the mass, in which he attempts to make everyone aware of the sacrament's healing power. But he's frustrated. Those most in need of anointing have been physically unable to get to church. Throughout the year, Father tries to minister to these infirm people in their homes, but he's the only priest at St. Mary's now, and his other responsibilities leave no time for regular home visits to the parish's shut-ins. What can he do?

• Lila is a parishioner at St. Peter's who claims to be a "healer," yet she has made no effort to have her ministry commissioned by the church. Father Joe has become concerned about Lila's actions because three parishioners have come to him in a state of distress, saying she told them they had "an evil spirit." Father feels that Lila is a loose cannon in the parish. What new disaster is she going to cause in the name of Jesus?

• John, who belongs to St. Anthony Parish, has just learned he has diabetes. Frantic with worry, he attends a faith healing service that features a nationally known "healer" who's come to town for the weekend. She tells the audience that if they have enough faith, God *must* heal them. All they have to do is "claim their healing," stop taking medicine, and ignore any remaining symptoms of their illness. John knows he'll slip into a diabetic coma if he quits taking insulin, and he doesn't think he has enough "faith" to claim his healing. He leaves the service more distressed than when he arrived. Now, in addition to feeling like a physical failure, he feels like a spiritual one as well. Utterly demoralized, he quits going to mass. Members of his parish are concerned. What should they do?[1]

We who are members of the Body of Christ must begin to offer help to these wounded in our midst by caring for them ourselves. Lay and ordained, staff and volunteers, young and old — all of us must reach out to parishioners like those we've just described. This book tells how to do that without resorting to fanaticism. It explains how to bring sufferers into the presence of God, where they can be healed. As in the time of Jesus, the illnesses may be physical, emotional, spiritual or relational. Our God and savior wants to heal them all.

Before we can move into the subject of expanded healing ministry, we need to examine how the church currently cares for the sick within its parishes. Much of that care now centers on what officially is called *Pastoral Care of the Sick: Rites of Anointing and Viaticum*. This sacrament, anointing of the sick, is little known, underused, controversial and in need of support.

The Mystery Sacrament

Five sacraments are well known to Catholics because they *experience* them. Babies get baptized during Sunday masses; most mass-goers receive the eucharist every week; everyone retains deeply felt recollections of the sacrament of reconciliation (penance) even if its use has drastically waned; adults remember the moment they were confirmed; and weddings occur weekly. Most Catholics know that a sixth sacrament — holy orders — is the rite for becoming a priest.

The remaining sacrament is a mystery to many unless someone says "last rites." Then a flash of recognition crosses people's faces. A few remember its old name: extreme unction. Everyone envisions a priest rushing to a dying person's bedside. Prior to the Second Vatican Council, their impressions were accurate. For centuries, extreme unction (literally "last anointing") was a sacrament for the dying, not the living.[2] It focused on spiritual preparation for meeting the Lord face to face.[3] This spiritual aspect evolved into a belief that "to die immediately after extreme unction guaranteed an unimpeded journey to God."[4]

The Second Vatican Council made dramatic changes regarding this sacrament, changes which have not been fully implemented or understood. Vatican II adopted a new rite of anointing of the sick in order to reflect its renewed awareness of the commission that Jesus gave his disciples: to continue the healing ministry he had begun in his day. Its document for pastoral care of the sick acknowledges this commission in the introduction:

> The Lord himself showed great concern for the bodily and spiritual welfare of the sick and commanded his followers to do likewise. This is clear from the gospels and above all from the existence of the sacrament of anointing, which he instituted and which is made known in the Letter of James.[5]

The above mentioned passage from the Letter of James is a key for the anointing of the sick. It shows how Jesus' disciples lived out his commission to the church during its earliest days:

> Is there any one of you who is sick? He should call the church
> elders, who will pray for him and pour oil on him in the name
> of the Lord. The prayer, made in faith, will save the sick man:
> the Lord will restore him to health (Jas 5:14–15a, *TEV*).

"Restore to health." How many people know that a sacrament exists through which they can experience this? How many know that healing is something they should expect to experience through the "church elders"? How many know this sacrament can be used for physical *and* emotional healing?[6] How many know that Jesus told his followers to fight against the evil of *all* suffering, including the suffering caused by illness? This last point flies in the face of the widespread belief that illness is God's will, a chastisement, or a test he sends to those who love him. This folk legend smothers all thought of a loving, compassionate God who sent his Son into the world to *heal* it, not make it sick. If illness *is* God's will, then medical care wars against that will, and so does anointing of the sick.[7] That's absurd, of course, but it highlights the error of nearly a thousand years of church teaching.

Pastoral Care of the Sick discredits this long standing attitude:

> Suffering and illness have always been among the greatest prob-
> lems that trouble the human spirit . . . . Part of the plan laid out
> by God's providence is that we should fight strenuously against
> all sickness and carefully seek the blessings of good health, so
> that we may fulfill our role in human society and in the church.[8]

The fact that few people know and make use of this part of our heritage reveals what a mystery this sacrament has become. It tells us we need to revive a healing ministry that Christ instituted.

The Neglected Sacrament

The church teaches that Christ is truly *present* in the sacraments. They do not merely mimic what Jesus did 2,000 years ago. Instead, they make Christ literally *here* today through us, his followers. Anointing of the sick exists to make Christ present to Christians in the midst of their sickness. When he becomes real to them in their need, much healing occurs. Evil is defeated. They experience new wholeness, as Jesus' words come to life. "I have come so that they may have life and have it to the full" (Jn 10:10).

Few can experience fullness of life if they are doubled over with arthritic pain, addicted to alcohol, or paralyzed by memories of childhood sexual abuse. To observers of this suffering, Jesus' promise of fullness of life seems like, at best, a promise of happiness in heaven or, at worst, a bad joke. The problem doesn't lie with the sick, but with the Body of Christ. People's needs for healing are going unmet because pastoral care to the sick is woefully inadequate in the church today.

This neglect is so severe that it goes unrecognized. With the threat of priestless Sundays on the rise, people know they're in danger of being deprived of ready access to the sacrament of the eucharist. How many of these same people know they're *already* deprived of full use of the sacrament of anointing of the sick? Like a starving child who no longer clamors for food, few people seek ready access to healing ministry in their faith communities.

Who's to blame? Are there any ogres we can point fingers at? We don't think so. When this ministry was confined to preparation for death, no one knew they were neglecting a key task of Jesus, who came into the world to heal the sick and save humanity. Now that the church has regained the vision given her by Christ, parish priests are too overextended to give the pastoral care to the sick which the Second Vatican Council envisioned. Time pressures reduce priests' personal contact with hurting parishioners to such a minimal level that they have little chance to minister to their needs.

Traditionally, hospital chaplains have made extensive use of the anointing of the sick, yet fewer and fewer hospitals have resident priest chaplains. Those that still exist are badly handicapped by the endless interruptions of the hospital environment. Unless a priest covers a hospital 24 hours a day, seven days a week, some patients come and go before he can visit them. And when he does manage to reach patients, some of them panic because they think the offer of anointing means they're about to die.

Before anything can be done to remedy today's scarcity of healing ministry, people need to become aware of the original intention of the anointing of the sick and what a difference it can make in their lives. This will not be easy because many misunderstandings exist about this sacrament. Even theologians and liturgists disagree among themselves.

The Controversial Sacrament

The basic disagreement surrounding the anointing of the sick arises from the fact that a sacrament is supposed to infallibly produce its effect. The bread and wine become the body and blood of Christ at every consecration. Every person is born into the kingdom of God at the moment of his baptism. The Holy Spirit always comes upon a confirmand when she is confirmed. But not everyone gets well when he receives the anointing of the sick. What, then, is the intended effect of this sacrament? Herein lies the heart of the controversy.

Beyond the first few centuries, the official church has waffled on the answer to this question. For almost a thousand years it said that the intended effect of anointing of the sick was to give the sufferer strength to bear his illness without losing faith, and to forgive his sins if he needed forgiveness. The church also said the sacrament was meant to prepare someone for entering into the glory of heaven. These teachings solved the dilemma of the sacrament infallibly achieving its intended effect, but in the process Jesus' commission to cure the sick became a forgotten piece of the good news.

The Second Vatican Council debated this issue and ended up returning the sacrament's emphasis to what it was in the first century: restoration of health. Following the lead of Vatican II, theologians and liturgists of recent times have tried to give a balanced view, but most are fearful of unequivocally asserting that healing is the intended effect of the anointing of the sick. Their misgivings are especially strong when they talk about physical healing. For example, liturgist Thomas Talley says:

> . . . the sacrament itself gives no assurance that [physical heal-ing] will be the outcome. In such a case, then, one may well wonder in what sense physical healing can be an *effect* of the sacrament. If healing occurs, is such a restoration of bodily health a proper consequence of the sacrament. . . ? Or, to con-sider all the possiblilities, does the will of God at times oper-ate within and through certain of the arcane procedures of the American Medical Association?[9]

The controversy surrounding the anointing of the sick has filtered down to the parish level. Pastors, religious educators, and others have been reluctant to promise people something that the sacrament might not deliver. If a priest offers anointing to a woman with cancer and says, "This will cure you!" and then she gets worse, what will happen to her faith? How will she then see all other sacraments? What will she think of her relationship with God? And what will she think of the priest and the church? The horrors of these possibilities are so vivid that the ministry of religious healing has nearly vanished from the face of parish life. Rather than promise anything, parish ministers feel it's safer to promise nothing.

We believe that the source of misunderstanding with this sacrament is the mistaken belief that religious healing is one more form of health care. Looking at it from that perspective, an appendicitis patient has two choices: surgery or anointing of the sick. Or maybe he wants both, much like surgery plus antibiotics. If medical care is the primary goal in healing ministry, then we who engage in this ministry are guilty of practicing medicine without a license.

We spend an entire chapter (chapter 3) dealing with this concern. Here, we simply will say that when the instructions to the rite of anointing of the sick speak of "restoration of health," they cannot mean exactly what a physician means. To Jesus, "health" meant much more than the absence of sickness. It meant the wholeness of God. In fact, the word salvation comes from the Latin word *salus*, which means health! This highlights the fact that health and healing aren't minor matters in the life of the church. Rather, they are part of the very reason for the church's existence.[10]

Administered well, the sacrament of anointing of the sick always empowers a person to move closer to God's wholeness — to salvation. Something good always happens when this rite is done well. But poorly given, it will not produce its maximum effect. Today that's almost the norm in parish ministry because this is a sacrament that cries out for support.

The Sacrament in Need of Support

Father Paul could offer pastoral care to residents of a nearby nursing home only once a month, yet the residents needed frequent, loving support. So five parishioners committed themselves to minister at the home on a weekly basis, bringing communion to those who wanted it and spending time with people who rarely had other visitors.

When Father made his monthly visit, the lay ministers joined him. He celebrated mass for the ambulatory patients, then he and the ministers visited the rooms of those Catholics who were not able to come to mass. Just before entering a room, the minister briefed him about the patient's condition and needs. If he was experiencing a medical or emotional crisis, the sacrament of anointing of the sick was administered. The presence of the lay minister greatly enhanced the experience. The patient already loved and trusted her, so she provided a comforting thread of continuity. The sacrament was given within the love of a small faith community. Within this context it became more than a mechanical ritual. It became a celebration of God's loving, intimate care. Jesus became real to the hurting person.

This is the kind of support anointing of the sick needs in order to achieve its maximum effect. A look at the other six sacraments makes it apparent that they, too, require support. Baptisms, marriages and confirmations take place in front of the assembly gathered at mass and involve the efforts of more than the priest. Celebrants of the eucharist are supported by lectors, servers, ushers, choirs and eucharistic ministers. The sacrament of reconciliation is often celebrated in communal penance services. Jesus instituted *all* the sacraments to be celebrated within the faith community. This includes the sacrament of anointing of the sick.

> The sacramental act has no meaning if it is not in the context of the tender, loving care of a real community of faith . . . . What this says about the size and character of churches, communities of faith, is obvious . . . . [It suggests] that at least we can provide for the simple training of large numbers of persons for visiting the sick.[11]

Vatican II's new rite of pastoral care affirms the faith community's responsibility to complement the priest's role in this rite. It allows and even exhorts the laity to be a part of the celebration of anointing of the sick: "This ministry is the common responsibility of all Christians, who should visit the sick, remember them in prayer, and celebrate the sacraments with them."[12]

Support does not mean replacing the priest's role in this sacrament. Some people fear that if the non-ordained become involved in healing ministry, the distinction between ordained and non-ordained will become blurred. This competitive attitude sets up a no-win situation. It robs people of the care they deserve from the church, burdens priests with the whole task of ministering to the sick, and excludes those who may have profound gifts to offer to this little used yet much needed ministry of religious healing.

Instead of thinking competitively, we must begin thinking cooperatively. All members of the Body of Christ must begin to bring God's healing touch to hurting people. That's why this book has been written: to give people both the vision and the tools they need to continue a ministry begun by Jesus, then entrusted to us, his followers.

Two Spiritualities

*What type of spirituality can meet the needs of
hurting people — Jesus-and-me, or Christ/we?*

Lila's tearful appearance took Leo by surprise. They had last talked
when she phoned to announce that God had given her a healing
ministry and that she was to work with Leo. When he said this
needed further discernment and recommended she receive training
to develop her gifts, Lila became enraged. Calling him a godless,
secular humanist, she slammed down the receiver.

The Lila who sat before Leo now was a shaken shadow of the
person who had once pronounced him godless. Since that original conversation, she had visited many local prayer groups and performed healings in their meetings. She had also invited people to
come to her home for further prayer. Her powerful personality attracted a number of followers, who looked on her as their spiritual
leader.

Then one evening Lila met Henrietta, an overweight woman
who had a severely infected hand. In an effort to help Henrietta
with her infection, two women invited her to join them at a healing
session in Lila's home. When it became Henrietta's turn for prayer,
Lila extended her right hand over her. Ignoring the prayer request,
Lila's hand trembled as she proclaimed that Henrietta had an evil
spirit of gluttony, from which she needed deliverance and inner
healing. Lila announced that, without these prayers, the infection
could not be healed. With no further explanation, Lila launched
into a deliverance prayer, asking everyone present to join in casting
out Henrietta's "evil spirit of gluttony."

This was Henrietta's first experience of healing ministry, and it
terrified her. Sobbing uncontrollably, she said she wanted to leave.

This only caused Lila to intensify her efforts, saying this resistance came from the evil spirit. Finally, Henrietta's two friends had sense enough to help her leave. She continued sobbing all the way home. "I always knew I was a bad person," she said, "but not that bad."

At home, Henrietta locked herself in her bedroom while the friends attempted to explain to her husband what had happened. He became furious, ordered them out of the house, and told them to stay away. For two days Henrietta refused to come out of her room or allow anyone in because she said she had an evil spirit and others might "catch it."

Lila might have continued her style of ministry if it hadn't been for what happened next: Henrietta's husband threatened to sue. This got Lila's attention. Fear brought her to Leo's door, motivated to look at ministry in a different light.

Although a Catholic, Lila had been attending a non-denominational charismatic prayer group where she "received her gift of healing." While there, she also learned a highly individualistic approach to Christianity, sometimes called a Jesus-and-me spirituality.

Jesus-and-me spirituality contrasts so sharply with incarnational spirituality, which we'll call Christ/we, that it has led to serious conflicts within Christianity. We believe it forms a tragic wall that separates countless followers of Christ from one another. Nowhere is this wall more apparent than in healing ministry. If we want to deal effectively and lovingly with those who turn to us for help (whom we call "supplicants"), we need to see how these two forms of spirituality impact our ministry to them.

Jesus-and-Me Spirituality

A Jesus-and-me spirituality focuses exclusively on the individual's relationship with Christ. Although fellowship with other Christians is seen as necessary for personal spiritual growth and for performing certain religious tasks, the church is just a human institution. The Spirit does not dwell or operate in the church as such, only in the individual. Because in this approach the church has no divine dimension, membership is optional and is not something willed by God. Here, then, the church is merely a voluntary association of individuals, each of whom has a personal relationship with Jesus. It is important to note that no single Christian faith teaches all aspects of a Jesus-and-me spirituality. This description is a composite of many affiliations.

A Jesus-and-me view of the church shapes members' understanding and practice of ministry. For them, God alone directly calls a person to a ministry, without the mediation of any person or group. Therefore the call does not depend upon being commissioned by any authority in the church. Since the Spirit does not reside in the church, it is incapable of verifying the authenticity of an individual's call. The person called, with the personal help of the Spirit, makes this discernment without the help of others.

Lila's Jesus-and-me view of the church caused distortions in her ministry. Excessive individualism put her in an isolated spiritual position and exposed her to the danger of self-deception. Only she could authenticate her call; only she could critique the quality of her ministry.

Lila adopted a take-it-or-leave-it approach to others' discernment. Instead of seeking feedback in her original phone call, she simply announced what she thought God had told her. Her fascination with "having a ministry" deafened her to Leo's caution to test the authenticity of the call and to develop her gifts. Since, in her mind, the church played no part in issuing her call, the church had no right to dabble in discernment. Lila was accountable only to God.

The Church Is the Body of Christ

St. Paul's and Lila's views of church would have collided head-on after his experience on the road to Damascus. "Breathing threats to slaughter the Lord's disciples" (Acts 9:1), Paul was traveling to Damascus to arrest any Christians he could find. Suddenly, however, Christ appeared to him in a blinding light that dropped him to the ground.

> "Saul, Saul, why are you persecuting me?" "Who are you, Lord?" he asked, and the answer came, "I am Jesus, whom you are persecuting" (Acts 9:4–5).

Neither Paul's life nor that of the entire early church was the same after that encounter. Paul thought he was persecuting the followers of Jesus, but Jesus' words revealed that the one who spoke to him was now more than an individual. He was the Total Christ. The Total Christ — then and now — is Jesus the Lord, living in glory with the Father in heaven, with all believers joined to him in an intimate way.

To explain to converts his understanding of the revelation on the road to Damascus, Paul used the image of the human body: "Now you are the Body of Christ, and each one of you is a part of it" (1 Cor 12:27, *NIV*).

A footnote in the *New Jerusalem Bible* further explores this:

> The words spoken by the Lord at Paul's conversion . . . imply that Christians are identified with the risen Christ. In Paul's writings, Christians are bodily united with the risen body by baptism and the eucharist, which make them parts of Christ's body, united in such a way that he and they together form the Body of Christ" (1 Cor 12i).

Modern English dampens the impact of Paul's profound vision because the word "body" carries several meanings, such as the human body or a group of people (e.g., a legislative body). A Jesus-and-me spirituality sees the Body of Christ as a society with a common way of life whose founder was Jesus. But if this were true, then we would be the Body of *Christians*.[1]

An incarnational, Christ/we spirituality sees the Body of Christ as the actual physical presence of the risen Lord, comprised of all Christians bonded to Christ as their head. "Just as each of us has various parts in one body, and the parts do not all have the same function: in the same way, all of us, though there are so many of us, make up one body in Christ" (Rom 12:4–5a). This spirituality sees the church as a living organism into which the Holy Spirit breathes life. By baptism and faith a person becomes so identified with Christ that together they become one being, even though each retains his or her unique individuality. Because the church is the Total Christ, we must love her as we love Christ himself.

We are the fullness or completion of Christ! Without us, Christ would not be whole or total: "You know, surely, that your bodies are members making up the Body of Christ" (1 Cor 6:15a, *JB*). Each Christian is joined to Christ so intimately as to become one body — one total Person. That unity also encompasses other Christians. Therefore Christians are bonded to one another as intimately as the parts of the human body. "All of us, though there are so many of us, make up one body in Christ, and as different parts we are all joined to one another" (Rom 12:5).

The church, then, is more than an association of believers in Christ. We, as Christians, are not free to belong to the church or not, as it meets our needs. We are Christian precisely *because* we belong to the Body of Christ, the church.[2] God calls each of us into intimacy with him, but that intimacy could not exist without others. The idea of a triune God does not spring, unbidden, into a nonbeliever's head. Instead, the tenets of our faith, the words of sacred scripture, the eucharist and countless other blessings have come to us through our faith community, a community which continues to hand on and teach us about the depth and breadth of God's revelation. We *need* the Church.

A Christian's belief in independence from the Body of Christ is comparable to, say, an American's fantasy of independence from other citizens. Let an earthquake strike and the self-reliant person quickly discovers that more than his dishes have been shaken up. His electricity off, his home becomes a cold cave, his food rots in the refrigerator. Suddenly the truth becomes apparent: independence is a proud delusion. So too with faith. It can only be born, nurtured, and reach maturity within the church. We are Christian *because* we belong to the Body of Christ.

Some writers use strong language to stress this point. For instance, theologian John C. Haughey states:

> The Spirit came to the community, not to individuals. Though the risen one appeared to individuals before he sent his Spirit, ever since this moment, individuals receive the Spirit and the presence of the risen one, only through the community. . . . Even the audacious singularity of Paul, the Apostle, had to await the ministrations of Ananias before he could be baptized and filled with the Holy Spirit. The loner who claims he is being led by the Spirit is a liar.[3]

Giving up the illusion of independence is difficult without a model of church that makes sense. Jesus offers the model of the vine and the branches:

> I am the vine, you are the branches. Whoever remains in me, with me in him, bears fruit in plenty; for cut off from me you can do nothing. . . . You did not choose me, no, I chose you; and I commissioned you to go out and to bear fruit, fruit that will last" (Jn 15:5, 16).

In other words, God has chosen us for a purpose: to bear fruit, to be the extension of Christ in time and space now that he has ascended into heaven. If we sever ourselves from the vine — the Total Christ, the church — we are useless to God. "Anyone who does not remain in me is thrown away like a branch — and withers" (Jn 15:6a, *JB*).

This union of the individual with Christ and with all other Christians is organic. The branch is not glued on to the stock; the hip is not sewn onto the pelvis. Together, the branches and the stock make up one plant. Human limbs and organs make up one person. This means any Christian action comes totally from Christ *and* totally from the minister, just as grapes produced by the vine come totally from the branches and totally from the stock. In incarnational, Christ/we ministry, the word "my" does not exist because all ministry belongs to the Total Christ. *Ministry — and healing — flow from the Body of Christ.*

Ministry Flows From the Body of Christ

Like it or not, we are all bonded together in Christ. Just as a fractured hip impacts the entire person and, thus, all parts of the body, so a wound to one Christian injures the Total Christ. This, in turn, injures every other Christian as well. "If one part if hurt, all the parts share its pain. And if one part is honored, all the parts share its joy" (1 Cor 12:26).

Like a human person, the church must grow to reach full stature. It needs food, water, and tender, loving care in order to achieve that growth. If a member is injured or becomes diseased, the whole body needs healing. Christ, as head of his body, organizes this growth, provides the nourishment needed and heals the diseased or injured member. "Under Christ's control the whole body is nourished and held together...and grows as God wants it to grow" (Col 2:19, *TEV*).

But Christ does not perform these functions apart from his total body. He is the organizing force, but he utilizes his members to nourish and to heal his body. In the physical body the mind needs the eyes, the arms, the hands to feed the body or to massage an aching muscle. Likewise, Jesus, the head of the body, utilizes physicians, nurses, psychologists, medicine, the sacraments and ministers to bring healing to an ailing member of his body.[4] When we lose sight of this truth, damage occurs in three areas.

1. The minister becomes a self-focused performer.

If a Jesus-and-me approach to ministry achieves its goal of healing, the minister may become an isolated "superstar." This, in turn, may distort and, finally, destroy genuine service to God and to humankind. In Lila's case, her preoccupation with "having" a ministry turned her into a performer rather than a minister. Henrietta was a stage prop for Lila's act. Henrietta's only importance was making Lila's ministry possible.

Because Lila believed that the Spirit dwelled solely within the individual, she had no choice but to be a "Lone Ranger." This left her ministry open to serious distortions. For example, she failed to establish rapport with supplicants. Without permitting Henrietta to tell her story, she could not reach a mutually acceptable agreement about ministry. Instead, she forced "her" ministry on her. In the absence of outside discernment from others, she placed excessive trust in unusual phenomena such as using her trembling hand to detect the presence of evil spirits. When things went badly, she blamed Henrietta.

2. The supplicant can be devastated.

A "superstar" can do a lot of damage. A gifted person like Lila may dramatically cure many people. This will attract a lot of attention and may draw a large following. But when dramatic cure is the goal, there are inevitable failures, and failures are an embarrassment to a superstar. The uncured supplicant looks like a giant weed in a formal English garden and must be disposed of quickly. In this hurried environment, disappointment is not handled responsibly. Often the supplicant is blamed for the failure. ("If you had enough faith, you would be healed.") Sometimes the damage is no more than disappointment. Sometimes, as in the case of Henrietta, the damage is devastating.

3. The ministry of religious healing is harmed.

In the long run, when healing ministry is not done within the Body of Christ, the greatest damage is to the very ministry of healing prayer itself. Unfortunately, in the public's mind — both Christian and non-Christian — the isolated superstar has become the standard image of the minister of healing prayer. The picture of flamboyant, weeping, claim-your-healing style "healers" has understandably made people suspicious of this entire ministry. An incarnational, Christ/we approach can bring healing into the realm of ordinary pastoral care.

Changing From Jesus-and-Me to Christ/We Spirituality

A badly shaken Lila had experienced the harm that can arise in the superstar form of healing ministry. The damage to Henrietta and the threatened lawsuit had caused her faith in God to waver. Overly confident that God was leading her directly, she had believed that she could do no wrong. "Where was God?" she cried to Leo. "Why did he let this happen to me? After people prayed over me and told me I'd received the gift of healing, I felt such power. I couldn't believe God would let anything bad happen. What went wrong?"

Leo's conversations with Lila convinced him that she was a gifted person who loved God. Buried beneath her fascination with healing lay a genuine desire to help hurting people. Her uncritical acceptance of a Jesus-and-me spirituality had led her into serious trouble and had robbed her ministry of its authenticity. Now she needed to adopt the communal, incarnational concept of church. She needed to discern what gifts God had given her, and to develop them in company with other Christians. She also needed to learn how to minister prayer for healing in a disciplined way.

Several things helped Lila in her struggles. First, she was strongly motivated to discover why things had gone badly for her. Secondly, as a "cradle Catholic," she had unconsciously absorbed an incarnational understanding of the church during most of her life. Finally, she had grown to love scripture during her association with the non-denominational prayer group. This love proved a big help because the teaching that the church is the Body of Christ is clearly scriptural.

A burden was lifted from Lila's shoulders when she realized she was only one ingredient in healing ministry. It subdued her to realize she was only a *part* of an instrument used by the Lord in his ministry. But it was also a relief. She came to see that the ministry of healing prayer is Christ, the head, using a number of people to heal a member of his body. Lila's liberation came when she saw that she didn't have to be the messiah. She could reach out to hurting people within the safety and power of the Body of Christ. Even though this was a relief, paradoxically it placed more responsibility upon her.

She needed to become a fit instrument for Jesus to use; ineptness would hinder the work of Christ.

To develop into a mature minister of religious healing, Lila agreed upon a reading program plus weekly discussions with Leo plus enrollment in the Institute for Christian Ministries (ICM), an ecumenical, two-year training program designed to train Christians for team ministry. With the help of peers in the training program, she could discern what gifts God had given her. Then she could develop these gifts by study, training, and reflection upon her ministry.

Lila had acted independently for so long that it was humbling for her to be accountable to others. She had acquired attitudes that made it difficult for her to allow others to look at, reflect upon, make judgments about her ministry. But slowly, Lila blossomed in the warmth of her peers' affirmation of her gifts. They saw gifts and strengths in her that she was blind to. She told Leo she had never experienced such a loving, supportive community before. Her former followers had placed her on a pedestal for their own needs, but they had not esteemed her for her true self. The ICM group valued her enough to tell her the truth about herself, positive and negative. This experience revealed to Lila the blessing of the church's concern for the quality of ministry and for the well-being of its ministers.

Receiving Ministry From the Body of Christ

Understanding the church to be the Body of Christ changes the role of the supplicant. Ministers who see the church as the Body of Christ treat the recipient of ministry as a valued member of that body. He is an equal participant in the process of healing. This attitude counters the temptation to put the supplicant in an inferior position while elevating the minister's importance.

This temptation comes as much from the supplicant's attitude as from the minister's. Most of us tend to bring to healing ministry the attitude with which we approach physicians. They are the experts. We place our fragile bodies in their hands and take a passive role in treatment. The physician, with the help of other health care professionals, makes a diagnosis, selects a treatment plan and evaluates its effectiveness. The patient's role is to follow directions and fill out insurance forms.

Today a few voices in the health care professions are protesting this arrangement.[5] But even if what we've described is suitable for scientific medicine, it is inappropriate for the ministry of religious healing. A supplicant is not a patient, and a minister is not a physician. The supplicant, even in her role of seeking healing, is as much a member of the Body of Christ as are the ministers. Therefore, she must take an active role in her own healing (Chapter 8 discusses this).

The Role of the Institutional Church in Healing Ministry

Lila finally had to confront her feelings about the institutional aspects of the church. She had absorbed the non-denominational prayer group's teaching that these aspects were "man-made." This teaching ignored contrary biblical evidence that the institutional parts of the church are also the work of the Holy Spirit. For example, in the Acts of the Apostles the Holy Spirit spoke through the prophets and teachers of the Church at Antioch in choosing Barnabas and Paul as missionaries (Acts 13:2–3). When Jewish Christians challenged the ministry of Paul and Barnabas to the Gentiles and accused it of being unorthodox, the matter was submitted to the leaders in Jerusalem, who said, "It has been decided by the Holy Spirit and by ourselves not to impose on you any burden beyond these essentials . . ." (Acts 15:28).

Lila's resistance to the institutional church faded as she studied scripture passages about the church being the Body of Christ. She came to realize that, just as a marriage succeeds only if both partners care for each other, people can minister effectively only within a church they cherish. This means respect for authority and love for the people of God. Without these, ministers use up their emotional energies wrestling with anger and distrust. They also resist learning from members of the Body of Christ, especially from its leaders. In the long run, this robs them of competence and community.

If all ministry belongs to the entire Body of Christ, then the institutional church must involve itself in that ministry. It needs to discern who is called to ministry, organize the training, and supervise the ministry itself. Christ as head uses ordained ministers to organize the many ministries of his body. They must be organized because no one of them can stand alone. Ordained ministers, on behalf of the total Body of Christ, have the duty to examine other ministers to ensure that each one demonstrates an ability to serve the Body of Christ in ways that will build it up. Each ministry must be guided by teaching and policies if the Body of Christ is to flourish.[6]

The role of ordained ministers is more nurturing than is sometimes thought. Not only do the ordained evaluate and supervise ministry, but they foster it as well. At this point in history, the ministry of religious healing desperately needs the attention of the church's ordained ministers! It cries out for more initial and continuing training opportunities. It needs the encouragement and support of wise leaders in discovering the right persons to exercise healing ministry.

Healing Ministry Is Ordinary

In a Jesus-and-me approach to ministry, supplicants often wait until a superstar healer rides into town promising healing for all who have faith. The superstar usually moves quickly from town to town, leaving a giant hole where long term and follow-up ministry should exist. This is one of the most serious drawbacks of the ministry given by itinerant healing evangelists. After a healing prayer session, people are left on their own. Questions remain unanswered and residual problems unsolved. Is it any wonder, then, that many revival-type healings end up being fleeting successes?

Healing that takes place within the Body of Christ is "ordinary." Supplicants receive as much support as they do in other types of pastoral care, for example, counseling, instructing, comforting. They can pray with parish-based ministers on a regular basis for as long as needed. The ministers are accessible and come to know — and love — the supplicant.

For example, our original supplicant, Henrietta, finally received "ordinary" help for her problems. First she received medical care for her infected hand. After she had recovered, two new friends who were experienced ministers of religious healing invited her to join a social group they belonged to. Henrietta refused. Her already low self-esteem had been severely damaged by her misunderstanding of deliverance and inner healing, and she believed she was a "bad sinner" who might harm the group. The friends listened, then later asked her to read a book which explained inner healing and deliverance in a sound, non-sensational way.

Over time, the friends discussed these topics with Henrietta and reassured her she had been poorly ministered to. They emphasized that the need for inner healing or deliverance did not mean a person was bad. Finally, the friends prayed with Henrietta that she might recover from her experience of poor ministry. They did not pray for any other inner healing, since they judged her to be too vulnerable at that time. The friends' prayers seemed to alleviate Henrietta's anxiety; she joined the social group and returned to a normal life.

Through people like Henrietta's new friends, the risen Lord is present in every parish, in every church, in every place, for all time. The Father intended, through Christ's work, to recreate a universe damaged by sin. "He would bring everything together under Christ, as head, everything in the heavens and everything on earth" (Eph 1:10).

Because Christ's life on earth lasted less than forty years, his work of forging an entirely new creation had hardly begun at the time of his ascension. Now risen and ascended into heaven, Christ our head asks us, the members of his body, the church, to participate in completing his task of recreating the universe. As Lila discovered after two years of community-based study and prayer — alone, we can't succeed; together, we can't fail.

Summary: Comparing Two Spiritualities

	Jesus-and-Me	Christ/We
Church	a volunteer organization of believers, a man-made institution	the Body of Christ, of divine origin, instituted by Christ
Spirit	dwells only within the individual, *not* within any church	dwells in the individual *plus* in the church as a whole, the Body of Christ
Christ's presence	in the word (Bible) plus within each individual Christian	in the word, in the sacraments, plus in the fullness of *all* Christians united into one body with Christ as its head
Christians	individual believers in Christ	an extension of Christ in time and in place, incarnational

	Jesus-and-Me	Christ/We
Call to ministry	only by God, therefore no one else can discern or test the call nor critique the ministry	by God *plus* the Body of Christ, individual call authenticated and commissioned by the church after discernment
Discernment of God's will and of gifts	personal interpretation of scripture, personal prayer, physical phenomena, circumstances	personal prayer, scripture *plus* the help of the church through study, reflection, and training
Role of church leadership	preach the word, guide, direct the organization, as a human organization	foster, train, evaluate, and supervise ministry, speaking in the name of Christ
Common style of ministry	isolated, if successful can lead to superstar mentality, no outside discernment	team, ordinary, within the Body of Christ in a faith community, ministry flows from the Body of Christ
Role of supplicant	passive, no rapport with minister needed, below level of minister	active, has gifts as a part of Body of Christ, team *enables* the supplicant, equal participant

Chapter Three

What Is Health?

Health is the goal in healing ministry, but
what is the religious meaning of health?

David knew the headaches well. Each one started with a flash of light, the opening credits for an internal laser show. The light would then progress into continuous, pulsating, circular patterns, like ripples caused by a stone thrown into a pond. While these auras were going on, David was blind in the center of his vision. This made driving dangerous, yet whenever a "light show" struck, he knew he needed to go home immediately. The brain-pounding pain of a migraine was about to begin.

Once home, David would take a dose of the narcotic his doctor had prescribed for his headaches. Then he would go to bed, usually for two days, sometimes for three. The room had to be in total darkness because light stabbed his eyes like knives. The slightest noise caused waves of nausea to sweep over him. Just turning his head would make him throw up. Sometimes the pain even blotted out his memory of those two or three days.

After countless tests all proved negative, David's doctor said he had done everything he could. Since he could find no cause for the headaches, he regretted he could do nothing more than give David pain medication. "You'll have to learn to live with them," he told his dejected patient. The trouble was, these migraines were increasing in frequency — from three or four a year, they began to occur once a month, then every three weeks. At a loss of several days' work each time, David's sick leave had vanished by mid-year. His job was at risk due to his absenteeism, and his family life was beginning to suffer.

The Body as Machine

Different people might approach David's problem in different ways, depending on how they answered one basic question: What is health?[1] Some would answer like an auto mechanic responding to a broken transmission, looking at the body as a machine. When the body is a machine, then humans are nothing more than warm-blooded automobiles. Broken down people go to surgery, where their engines are taken apart so that the surgeon/mechanic can fix the part (say, a heart valve) or replace it with a new one. Medication for a fever can be compared to putting an additive into gasoline. A "formula" will fix everything. If it isn't fixed, then the correct formula hasn't been found.[2]

Just as some mechanics only do transmissions, some physicians only do eyes or hands or skin. This specialization arose when medicine allied itself with the budding science of chemistry. Scientists discovered germs, learned how to kill some of them, and liberated us from such dread diseases as smallpox, polio and typhus. What arrived with this liberation, however, was a single-cause theory of medicine: a disease like smallpox is caused by one particular germ. Find that germ, develop a vaccine, and — voila! — no more disease.

Alas, what may be valid with germs does not work with all ailments. Furthermore, the single-cause theory of medicine ends up separating a person into little pieces that act according to the laws of physics and chemistry. Nurses talk about the "tonsillectomy in room 632" or the "appendectomy in bed 4." This cold, almost cruel, detachment deals only with the sick part and not with the sick person. It is a natural offshoot of the need we all have to understand the world we live in. A tonsil is predictable and can be quantified; it sits in the throat, measures so-much by so-much, and can be removed if it becomes repeatedly infected. But the whole human person lying in a hospital bed — body, mind, and spirit — is *not* predictable. We can't deal with people as easily as we can deal with their parts. Therefore we focus our attention on parts instead of people.

Trouble comes when no broken part can be found. David approached his physician as he would have his mechanic, asking him to "fix" his migraines. Thorough exams revealed no underlying pathology such as a brain tumor. No pieces were "broken," no germs had taken up residency in David, yet his life was disintegrating. The only available treatment seemed to be taking pain pills, which dulled his mind, but not his pain.

Throughout recorded history, the medical community has seen millions of Davids and has struggled with how to treat them. During the past century physicians have begun to distinguish the differences between disease and illness. In the process, they've been able to see that curing and healing are not synonymous.

Disease vs. Illness, Curing vs. Healing

Physicians see *disease* as a malfunctioning of biological or psychological processes. They use the word "health" to indicate freedom from disease. For them, health is a static state, and disease is a departure from that state. Often they see healing as a return to the optimum static state designated by the word health.

Illness, on the other hand, is the *experience* of disease. It is created by a patient's or supplicant's *reaction* to disease. For instance, a man with undiagnosed high blood pressure has a disease, but until that fact is known, he does not have an illness. Once he becomes aware of his disease, he responds in a variety of ways, e.g., depression about the side-effects of medication, or fear that he might have a stroke. Society's reaction to his disease shapes his reaction as well. When his wife nags him about using salt, he feels angry. When his employer passes him over for a promotion because he's a health risk, he feels like a failure. Together, the man's reactions add up to illness.

According to physician and public health officer Eric Cassell, "disease is something an organ has; illness is something a man has."[3] This distinction impacts treatment and reveals the contrast between curing and healing. When doctors, therapists or religious healers conquer a disease, *it* is *cured*. In curing, what counts is the blood pressure, the fractured bone, the migraine headache. The *person* in whom the malady resides is irrelevant. On the other hand, when doctors, therapists or religious ministers *heal*, they heal a *person*. Looking beyond an isolated, nameless, faceless disease, they deal with a unique individual's total response to his or her disease.

In *Peace, Love and Healing*, Dr. Bernie Siegel writes:

> I certainly wouldn't give up any of the medical miracles that
> we twentieth-century doctors have available to us. That's why

I've remained a surgeon. But I can't help noticing that our power to *heal people* and their lives seems to have diminished as dramatically as our power to *cure diseases* has increased. This is because the knowledge of human nature that used to be the doctor's principal resource has been abandoned as irrelevant in an age of science. Science has become God, and separated itself from the patient.[4]

The Mind/Body Connection

The medical community now recognizes the link between mind and body. One impacts on the other and takes the question, "What is health?" beyond the realm of machinery. Psyche (mind) and soma (body) are as bonded together as the branches of a tree are to its trunk. Alone, neither survives because they are, in fact, one unit. The entire field of psychosomatic medicine exists to deal with this reality. Dr. Siegel makes a strong case for the impact of the mind on the body: "Feelings are chemical and can kill or cure. As a doctor I believe it's my responsibility to help my patients use them to cure and heal themselves."[5]

The chemicals Dr. Siegel refers to are peptide molecules which are made in the brain and the immune system.

[Peptide molecules] make feelings chemical and effect the link between psyche and soma. Endorphins, for example, are now thought to account for the placebo effect.... Pain relief really is "in the mind" — because that's where the endorphins are.[6]

After further describing the role of peptide molecules in health and healing, Dr. Siegel quotes neuropharmacologist Candace Pert of the National Institute of Mental Health:

I can no longer make a strong distinction between the brain and the body.... Indeed, the more we know about neuropeptides, the harder it is to think in the traditional terms of a mind and a body. It makes more sense to speak of a single, integrated entity, a "mindbody."[7]

Since the discovery of the impact of peptides on health, the number of physical diseases thought to have an emotional component has greatly increased. More than just stomach ulcers can occur in situations of high stress. Now physicians talk about the role the mind plays in cancer, in arthritis and, yes, in migraines.

David began to look at the connection between his migraines and his emotions when someone gave him a book titled *Migraine Relief.*[8] The book included a biofeedback finger band for measuring skin temperature. The band shows readers how warm or cool their fingers are. Cool skin temperature indicates tense muscles which, in turn, are often a prelude to a migraine attack.

In chapter 4 of *Migraine Relief,* author Robert Kohlenberg invites his readers to look courageously at *why* they are in a state of muscle tension. "You may learn something about yourself that you have not wanted to face before," he writes. "Your new awareness can lead to an awareness of psychological threats and disturbances that are in your environment."[9]

As David thought about the threats referred to by Dr. Kohlenberg, he realized the environment that disturbed him most was his interior one. He had never dared to look at the ravages of a childhood that had been filled with tragedy. "Let sleeping dogs lie," he said to himself whenever memories leapt into his conscious mind. The trouble was, the dogs were awake and barking, demanding attention for wounds that needed healing.

Intellectually, David knew his past. He knew his father had died in an automobile accident when he was an infant. One day three years later, his mother locked him in his room, stuffed rags at the bottom of his door to protect him from fumes, went downstairs to the kitchen, and turned on the gas oven. David's sisters found her body when they came home from school.

As if being orphaned weren't enough trauma, David and his sisters then were taken into an uncle's home where, over a period of the next fifteen years, two male relatives sexually abused the three of them. Their uncle never let them forget he had taken them in because of a sense of duty to their mother, not because he wanted them. These traumas left David with a myriad of profound, yet unrecognized, feelings: abandonment, anger, rejection, betrayal of trust, guilt, and low self-esteem.

The Body as Plant

No medical mechanic could give David a pill to make these issues — and headaches — go away. David needed a health specialist who could help him see his body as being connected to his mind, his spirit, *and* his relationships. Sometimes called holistic doctors, these specialists are like gardeners. When a plant wilts, the gardener examines its total surroundings: water, sunlight, soil conditions, insects, space, nutrients. He may talk to the plant and play soothing, classical music in order to create the ideal climate for growth and well-being. Like the gardener, the holistic physician deals with the whole patient in her environment.

In holistic medicine, health includes the way people feel and function, both physically and psychologically, as well as how they interact with their environment. *People* get sick, not just their livers and blood vessels, and these illnesses touch every aspect of their lives. Holistic specialists recognize the crucial need to treat Davids, not just migraines. In his case, a specialist would have three goals: remove the headaches, deal with the stresses or memories that are causing them, and restore any disrupted job or family relationships. Anything less would not be considered "health."

David had only one problem with a holistic approach to his health: the mere thought of examining his feelings about the past put him into a state of cold terror. This, in turn, spilled over into a generalized fear of his current life. One day he would be afraid to drive, the next he would be afraid to talk to his boss, the next afraid to go to work. His struggle to push down these multiple fears turned into a profound depression from which there seemed to be no escape, nor even any light of hope.

Finally David got so depressed that one day he said, "Wait a minute, there's got to be something else." He decided to change. He didn't decide to move forward. He just made a conscious decision to get out of pain. This decision led him into counseling where, over a period of the next year, he unearthed a profusion of feelings. First, he discovered he blamed himself for being an orphan because he was the only one home when his mother died. Subconsciously he played a number of mental "tapes" that kept this lie alive: "If I had been *better*, maybe I could have loved her more. If I had loved her more maybe she would have been OK, and then *I* would have been OK."

In counseling, David learned that his shattering experiences had left him with profoundly low self-esteem, an emptiness that said "you're not lovable." After unearthing many other feelings, he finally felt safe enough within himself to feel angry. He was angry at himself, his mother, his father, his uncle. David's anger also included identity problems. His anger at his uncle was partially due to the feeling that, "I was a part of their family, but I wasn't. I didn't have a name. I didn't belong anywhere. Who was I?" This swirl of subconscious messages, questions, and feelings had created constant muscle tension which, in turn, led to migraines.

The more David got in touch with his feelings, the rarer and less intense these migraines became. Everyone was delighted, but David began to see that although his malady had been *cured*, he still had an illness. Curing the disease of migraine headaches proved far easier than getting rid of the results of a shattered childhood. Within the safety of counseling and of a sexual abuse support group, David started to realize that his health extended beyond the state of the blood vessels in his brain. It touched the very fiber of his being. This realization led him into spirituality. Where was God in this situation?

The Miracle Worker

If we ask, "What is health?" from a spiritual viewpoint, we get a variety of answers, depending on whom we ask. Some think of religious healing as just a subdivision of healing in general, i.e., surgical healing, chemical (drug) healing, psychiatric healing, and religious healing. If this viewpoint is true, then we who engage in this ministry are "miracle workers" who do what physicians do, but without their resources. Instead of asking a doctor to intervene in a specific health problem, we ask God to intervene. We lose track of who we are: surgery with no knives! fillings with no dentists' drills! This is heady stuff. Is it any wonder that people who hold this view of healing can fall prey to a power trip?

The attitude of the few who pit themselves against the medical community lends credence to the accusation that some religious people practice medicine. Why take pills, they ask, when God will heal you directly? After seeing patients who have been left uncured by such ministry, some physicians come to judge all religious healers as dangerous charlatans. This creates a tragic separation between two valuable sources for healing.

The Religious Mechanic

Even if healing ministers avoid the trap of placing themselves in opposition to the medical community, it's easy to get locked into the message, "The only thing we can do is pray." In so doing, we miss exploring other options of care. Worse yet, within that single option of prayer we may focus on praying for only one symptom/problem.

Single-cause ministry focuses on only one problem and also tends to be preoccupied with one solution. Lila, for example, (in Chapter 2) saw disease as centered around evil spirits. Regardless of the request, she had one answer: deliverance. Ignoring other options in Henrietta's case, such as praying for the gift of courage to seek medical care, Lila plunged ahead with her predetermined treatment: casting out a devil.

Saddest of all, single-cause/single-solution religious "mechanics" miss seeing the person who stands before them. Lila failed to see *Henrietta* and her real needs. Like a physician who only sees a tonsil and surgery, she only saw obesity and deliverance. She had no idea what health is.

The Religious Meaning of Health and Healing

So, then, from a religious perspective, what *is* health? Throughout our lives we have been taught that Jesus was truly God and truly human. He was born with two natures: one human and one divine. We are born with one nature, a human one that is scarred by original sin. At baptism, however, something radical happens. St. Peter tells us we become "sharers of the divine nature" (2 Pt 1:4b, *NAB*).[10] Through no power of our own, we are given a share in God's divine nature! St. Paul describes it thus: "So for anyone who is in Christ, there is a new creation" (2 Cor 5:17a). St. John phrases it another way:

> My dear friends, we are already God's children, but what we shall be in the future has not yet been revealed. We are well aware that when he appears we shall be like him, because we shall see him as he really is (1 Jn 3:2).

In other words, through God's *gift* we acquire a share in the nature that Christ had by *right*. In baptism God transforms us so that now, although we still have only one nature, we are utterly transformed creatures.[11] Instead of being alienated by sin, God raises us to a new state of existence.

> The miracle of redemption is that God should change us, the unlovable ones, into the very likeness of his own Son, the Beloved. This transforming love is poured out in our hearts through the Holy Spirit who is given to us. It can only be a *giving* and *forgiving* love.[12]

This reality is fraught with potential for misunderstanding! Some people fear that being "sharers of the divine nature" is New Age, self-reliant thinking. They conclude that those who ascribe to this belief think they are their own god. But "man shares in the divine nature not in a divine but in a human way, consonantly with his nature as man."[13] Our radical dependency on God allows us to avoid delusions of grandeur and remain what we are called to be: co-heirs with Christ, adopted sons and daughters of God:

> [God marked] us out for himself beforehand, to be adopted sons, through Jesus Christ. Such was his purpose and good pleasure, to the praise of the glory of his grace, his free gift to us in the Beloved (Eph 1:5).[14]

Alas, Christianity often overemphasizes sin and deliverance instead of adoption into God's life and creativity. When this distortion occurs, salvation becomes nothing more than forgiveness of sins. This is a shadow of God's plan for us:

> The message of Jesus himself and of the early disciples was not just one of the forgiveness of sins, but rather was one of newness of life. . . . We who are saved are to have a different order of life from that of the unsaved.[15]

Sharing in God's divine nature is indeed a "different order of life!" Yet millions of Christians overlook this reality and instead preoccupy themselves with humanity's alienation from God. They spend so much spiritual and emotion energy dwelling on sinfulness and on the need for personal salvation that they ignore the new, divine life that Jesus won for humankind by his life, death, and resurrection. By getting stuck in the mire of personal sin, countless Christians neglect to work as co-creators with God through the Holy Spirit. They forget about their new life in Christ.

Theologian John C. Haughey states that Pentecost was the moment when God transformed humanity.

> The limitations that are imposed by each baptized Christian on the power of the Spirit. . .come not so much from our sinfulness, I suspect, as from our unwillingness to entertain the view of ourselves that God has of us.[16]

Jesus said "I have come so that they may have life and have it to the full" (Jn 10:10). *Life* epitomizes God's offer to the human family. According to scripture scholar Raymond Brown:

> God's greatest act of friendship to man was described in terms of man's receiving a share of God's life. The relation of this symbolism to that of becoming God's children is obvious.[17]

God's friendship with us will do what any friendship will do. It will transform us *to the extent* that we receive it. As with all friendships, we are free to accept or reject the offer, and we can accept it to different degrees. Because our "yes" to God's friendship almost always occurs one baby-step at a time, the transformation of our character advances at a pace which looks more like that of a snail than a gazelle. We grow gradually and partially into the fullness of God, and our slowness can cause us to lose heart. In the face of continuing sin we can forget our transformed nature. Our imperfections make it all too easy to drown in a sea of self-condemnation.

This despair is not God's will for us! He wants us to stay with him, to allow his friendship with us to permeate our total being until we become transformed into his own wholeness. In staying close to God, we will discover the answer to our original question of what is health. We will find that *health is the wholeness of God,* a wholeness we are called to when we become sharers in the divine nature. We grow *into* God's own health as we allow his friendship to transform our patterns of human behavior at every level of our being — mind, will, emotions, and even bodily functions.

The Spiritual Journey

Our snail's-pace transformation into God's health is called the spiritual journey, and it requires great tenacity and effort on our part. St. Paul had a keen awareness of the sort of exertion God asks of us:

Run so as to win! Athletes deny themselves all sorts of things. They do this to win a crown of leaves that withers, but we a crown that is imperishable . . . . What I do is discipline my own body and master it, for fear that after having preached to others I myself should be rejected (1 Cor 9:24b–25, 27, *NAB*).

Most of us shrink from Paul's strenuous effort, from submitting to the type of discipline he describes here. "That's for people like St. Peter or Mother Teresa," we protest. "I'm not that holy. I'm just ordinary. God doesn't expect me to do this." This thinking clashes with scripture, which does not divide Christians into the ordinary and the holy. If we allow ourselves the luxury of this "have" and "have-not" thinking, we will indeed make a feeble showing for our faith. A holy vs. ordinary mentality usually imprisons us in the "ordinary" category and rarely carries our journey with God beyond ourselves into service to the Lord through ministry to others.

In becoming sharers in the divine nature, we become sharers in Christ's mission to a broken world. We may not feel up to this task, but scripture assures us that, as brothers and sisters of Christ, we do more than is possible through our own human power and nature:

> The Spirit too comes to help us in our weakness, for, when we do not know how to pray properly, then the Spirit personally makes our petitions for us in groans that cannot be put into words (Rom 8:26).

In Christ, then, ministry extends beyond curing disease. It leads first us and then others into God's own health — the physical, emotional, spiritual, and relational wholeness of our triune God. Our call to the wholeness of God is a *lifelong* process that takes us beyond the vigor of a well-run physical machine, beyond the abundance of an environmentally sound, holistic garden. The *religious* meaning of health involves every dimension of our being. Our transformation will be complete when we see God face to face.

Summary: A Glossary of Terms

Disease: Something an *organ* has, a malfunctioning of biological and/or psychological processes.

Illness: Something a *person* has, the *experience* of disease. It is created by personal and social reactions to disease.

Curing: The overcoming of *disease* by intervention — physical, chemical, surgical or, sometimes, prayer. This is only one of the goals of the ministry of religious healing.

Healing: The overcoming of *illness* through treating the whole person — physically, emotionally, spiritually, and relationally. This is another goal of the ministry of religious healing.

Health: *Medical/Scientific:* The absence of disease.

             Religious: A sharing in the wholeness of God. Bringing a person into this reality is the ultimate goal of the ministry of religious healing. Becoming sharers in the wholeness of God is a lifelong process, called the *spiritual journey*, that involves every dimension of our being. Our transformation will be complete when we see God face to face.

Chapter Four

Ministry: "Here I Am, Send Me!"

Who is called to ministry, and what are its costs?

During the past decade "ministry" has become *the* buzz word within Catholicism. People throw it around with all the care and thought of a store clerk chanting "Have a nice day!" We can turn a meaningful word into thin gruel by overusing it, and this is one of those words. But the plus side of our recent love affair with "ministry" is that it indicates a changing theology:

> Until recently "ministry" was a Protestant word. Now it de-scribes a new situation in the Roman Catholic Church where more and more people want to be, claim to be ministers.... Church ministry expanding throughout the world suggests that the Holy Spirit is intent upon a wider service, a more diverse ministry for a church life that will be broader in quantity and richer in quality.[1]

The root meaning of ministry is service, a vague word if ever there was one. We ministers of religious healing need to understand our task more clearly than just to say we're "serving" or "ministering."

Called *and* Sent

Today's ministry continues the mission given to Jesus 2,000 years ago by his Father. According to theologian Richard McBrien, this involves first a calling, then a sending:

> The church is first called and then *sent*. In other words, the church is a community, or an assembly with a *mission*. The mission of the church is similar to that of Jesus Christ himself.[2]

47

In short, the church — and our participation in it — does not exist for the sake of our being cozy little Christians, called together into a holy huddle for the sake of our own personal salvation. Instead, the church exists to carry on the task given to Jesus by the Father.

Imagine our present fate if Jesus had regarded his call from the Father as simply being for his own spiritual benefit. At the Jordan River John would baptize him, then the Holy Spirit would descend on him like a dove, and a voice from heaven would say, "You are my Son, the Beloved; my favor rests on you" (Lk 3:22, JB). After that, Jesus would return home to Nazareth and resume his job as a carpenter. He would worship in the synagogue every sabbath and sometimes even journey to Jerusalem to offer sacrifice in the Temple. Whenever he would think back on his calling at the Jordan River, he'd say to himself, "What a great experience that was!" And after dying a natural death at the age of 75, everyone would say with great approval, "This was a holy man."

In the above scenario, Jesus assuredly would enjoy all the blessings of heaven, but he would rattle around there by himself because none of us could be saved. Thanks be to God, he realized his experience at the Jordan was a twofold call: an invitation into an ever deeper relationship with the Father and, then, a summons to serve. What was true 2,000 years ago remains true today: our first call *always* leads to the second, which sends us forth to minister to a wounded world. At the Last Supper, we see evidence of Jesus' awareness of his *and* our mission:

> I have revealed your name to those whom you took from the world to give me. . . . I have given them the teaching you gave me, and they have indeed accepted it . . . . (Jn 17:6, 8, 18).

So we who profess to be Christian need to accept the fact that being sent forth is an integral part of our reason for being followers of Christ. But to whom is God sending us? What does he want us to do? The answers to these questions depend on understanding that ministry means more than one thing.

Commissioned Versus Non-Commissioned Ministry

In religious healing, ministries can blur together. Once people have gained some experience in ministry, they often use their skills in a variety of situations such as praying with sick neighbors or working pastorally with parishioners who are in grief. With no special commissioning by the church, many people engage in broad Christian ministry, i.e., they minister to others in the name of Jesus. This is good.

Trouble arises when someone like Lila (Chapter 2) assumes her personal "success" in healing means that *God* has directly appointed her to a specific ministry. Egos swell, and people get hurt. Christ works through his Body, and that Body includes church leaders who bear responsibility for discerning, organizing, and supervising a variety of ministries. They have been empowered by the Body of Christ to commission others who are qualified for a specific healing ministry. This process of discernment averts countless problems and keeps everyone grounded in humility. Once we know the difference between commissioned and non-commissioned ministry, we can move on to looking more closely at how Jesus ministered to others. What did he say? What did he do? What was his focus?

The Kingdom of God

Jesus often referred to his mission as being one of bringing forth the kingdom of God. Christian scriptures frequently use the term kingdom: "The time is fulfilled, and the kingdom of God is close at hand. Repent, and believe the gospel" (Mk 1:15).

Today God calls us and sends us to help bring forth his kingdom. The most concise description we found to explain the kingdom of God comes from Thomas O'Meara's *Theology of Ministry*:

> In the phrase kingdom of God, "kingdom" is a word for the loving, active plan of God in history. . . . God's gracious plan transforms and challenges all it touches.[3]

An important word here is *active*. Jesus actively showed people what he meant when he proclaimed "the kingdom of God is close at hand." One way he fulfilled his mission to reveal the "loving, active plan of God" was through his healing ministry. Whenever he healed someone, he basically said, "This *is* the kingdom of God."

Jesus defended healing as an integral part of his mission. When challenged by his religious authorities because of his acts of healing, he responded by saying he was doing the work of God:

In all truth I tell you, by himself the Son can do nothing; he can do only what he sees the Father doing: and whatever the Father does the Son does too (Jn 5:19).

Today our ministry of religious healing is both an expression *and* an extension of Jesus' ministry. Healing moments make us aware that the kingdom of God is here, *now*, today. But one look at the pain that persists in the world shows us that the kingdom has yet to reach its fullness. To bring about God's "loving, active plan," God asks us to work with him. He calls us to be his co-workers, co-creators in making his dream come true. The task given to us, the church, is to be a clear channel of God's own self into a hurting world. As St. Francis of Assisi prayed: "Lord, make me a channel of your peace. . . . "

Today we could use an energy analogy for being channels of God's peace. For thousands of years, a huge oil source existed at Alaska's North Slope, but it remained useless without some means to bring it to the world. Now the oil flows through a pipeline and fuels automobiles and furnaces in countless cities and towns. Each of us is like a section of the Alaska pipeline, welded together into one piece, one body, so that God's powerful love can flow through us, bringing his kingdom "to all nations." We ourselves do not directly bring forth the kingdom; we don't create it. Instead we form a vital link between God and the world.

In the Footsteps of Jesus

On paper the idea of being co-creators sounds good. In reality the dream of helping to bring about the kingdom of God looks more like a nightmare. We listen to news reports of starvation in the midst of plenty. We meet adult after adult who was sexually abused as a child. We see the indictment of a corrupt government official on the six o'clock news. In the face of this pervasive evil, we just want to crawl into bed, curl into a fetal position and say, "Go away, world. I'm too puny for this task."

Jesus encountered the same evil 2,000 years ago, although the details differed. His society was well acquainted with starvation, sexual sin and government corruption. He came into the world precisely *because* it was as polluted as a toxic waste dump. He came because, in spite of everything, he loved it unconditionally. And he said "yes" to paying a price for that love.

During his temptation in the wilderness, Jesus reversed Adam and Eve's "yes" to Satan when he said "no" to the quick-fix, power-oriented ways of evil. His desert "yes" to the longer, humbler ways of the Father finally led to his death on the cross. Good Friday epitomizes the cost of ministry, and God asks each of us what price we are willing to pay. Few of us are asked to pay with our lives, but all of us are asked to carry the cross of ministry, to go out of our way each day to care for a wounded world.

> If anyone wants to be a follower of mine, let him renounce himself and take up his cross and follow me (Mt 16:24).

Carrying a cross has never been in style. According to Father John Shea,

> Taking up the cross means extending love to all people and enduring whatever suffering this endeavor might entail. There is that unknown "whatever." Like all unknowns, it is frightening. . . . Christians plead, "Bring us not to the test." No bravado there. Christians want to follow Jesus; but taking a clue from Peter, they want to do it "at a distance" (Lk 22:54). . . . When faced with the burden of the cross, . . . they wonder why they got involved in a way of life that demands so much? Perhaps there's a back door in the garden of Gethsemane.[4]

The gospels show that Jesus' way of the cross started long before the garden of Gethsemane. Desperate crowds hounded him (Mk 1:45, Lk 4:42); during his public ministry he was literally homeless with only the bare essentials of life (Lk 9:57–58); he didn't even have the approval of his own people (Lk 4:24,28–30; Lk 23:13–25). We can get the jitters when we consider the specifics of what Jesus' example may mean for us personally.

People who do decide to "deny themselves" and "take up their cross" can expect to pay a price in at least two ways:

1. The sacrifice of time and energy. If we believe Father Shea when he says that "taking up the cross means extending love to all people," we can anticipate that bringing this love to others will cost us time and consume physical, emotional and spiritual energy. Are we willing to *make* time for ministry? Can we say yes to using our precious stamina to bring Christ to a wounded, often ungrateful, world?

Our first expenditure of time and energy must be spent getting trained and educated to do effective ministry. Jesus faced this requirement, and so must we. The finding of Jesus in the Temple suggests that at the age of twelve he thought he was ready for ministry: "Did you not know that I must be in my Father's house?" "All those who heard him were astounded at his intelligence and his replies," but he was not yet ready for the ministry which the Father had planned for him. So he returned home to Nazareth with Mary and Joseph, where he "increased in wisdom, in stature, and in favor with God and with people" (Lk 2:49, 47, 52).

Every diocese has programs of training to prepare people for ministries. Students sacrifice hours, days and months to ready themselves to serve the Lord. Spiritual formation is a key ingredient in training programs because ministry is more than a task, and effective ministers are more than good job performers. They embody the words of St. Paul: "I am alive; yet it is no longer I, but Christ living in me" (Gal 2:20a). Those who "live in Christ Jesus the Lord" (Col 2:6a, *NAB*) succeed because people see and experience God through them. Conversely, ministers who focus on tasks or self-fulfillment fail:

> Our ministry will fall short of its desired effect unless we are faith-filled people; unless, in our own lives and ministry, we reflect the Lord and all his lovable qualities. People must see in us his love and mercy, his understanding and compassion.[5]

We cannot "reflect the Lord" unless we know him. To be faith-filled people, we must develop a vivid, personal relationship with Jesus, a relationship we *experience* at a felt level of our being. Jesus said, "I call you friends, because I have made known to you everything I have learned from my Father" (Jn 15:15b). He longs for the same friendship with us that he had with his disciples, one that has the normal ups and downs of any friendship but grows ever-deeper with each passing year. Ministry arises from the depths of this one-to-one relationship with Jesus.

When we are faith-filled people, we begin to think as God thinks because "we are those who have the mind of Christ" (1 Cor 2:16b). This is the essence of Christ/we, incarnational theology in ministry. It does not win any popularity contests in our task-oriented society or even in some parish communities. But as St. Paul said: "Do not model your behavior on the contemporary world, but let the renewing of minds transform you, so that you may discern for yourselves what is the will of God — what is good and acceptable and mature" (Rom 12:2).

A bigger sacrifice of time and energy lies beyond training because ministry continues for the rest of our lives. When Jesus said, "My food is to do the will of the one who sent me, and to complete his work" (Jn 4:34), he was describing his goal in life — doing God's will by completing the task the Father had started but not yet finished. The task was transformation of all creation, including the hearts and minds of every human being, and it *still* is not completed. God calls us to go forth in and with Christ and work toward that goal.

Are we willing to pray weekly with a woman who has been abandoned by her husband, or listen to a co-worker's story of pain? Opportunities for ministry rarely fit into our idea of a perfect day. Extending love to all people begins with making that love a time and energy priority.

2. *The price of holiness.*   Deeper costs of ministry lie beneath time sacrifices. God calls us to personal conversion, to reach our full potential as humans. This means becoming holy by living in total union with Christ.

Holiness always leads us to an experience of our spiritual poverty before God. We say "Lord, I am not worthy to receive you — or serve you." Worst of all, we even experience our sinfulness in ministry.The natural inclination in the face of this reality is to say "no" to ministry. Let God find someone who's holier, more adequate. With feelings of false humility we echo the words of Moses: "O Lord, please send someone else to do it" (Ex 4:13, *NIV*). But God didn't let Moses off the ministerial hook, and he doesn't let us off either. *Worthiness* is not the qualification test for ministry, *willingness* is.

When we serve God in spite of our unworthiness, we can count on several results: 1) *In* and *through* ministry, he will show us levels of spiritual impoverishment within ourselves that we never suspected existed. 2) That revelation will help us grow in holiness. 3) We will come to know that God is with us even in our mistakes. As we stay close to him, we will encounter God's infinite power to turn our mistakes and failings into something glorious for the kingdom of God.

Holiness is painful because it involves compassion. A heart of compassion will show us that the kingdom of darkness still strives to keep the world nailed to a cross. We encounter that darkness if we are willing to join people in their pain. If we say no to this form of holiness, then blindness and indifference will allow us to stand in the presence of pain without wincing. Just as brick walls have no feelings, neither will we if we surround our hearts with a protective layer of hardness. God wants to give us his heart of compassion so that we can bring love and healing where now we find hatred and pain.

Some ministers confuse compassion with phony cheerfulness. They attempt to jam artificial comfort down the throats of grieving supplicants by using words of hollow cheer. Their platitudes add up to withdrawal from another's pain. Imagine Jesus' response in the Garden of Gethsemane if his apostles had stayed awake and said "Don't worry, everything will be alright" as his sweat became like drops of blood falling to the ground! This type of emotional aloofness might have stung him even more than did their sleeping. What Jesus needed in Gethsemane was someone to *join* him in his suffering, not talk him out of it. He still needs that type of person today. Compassion heals people because it replaces isolation with hope. (For more on hope, see Chapter 9.)

Becoming the person God wants us to be will lead many to conclude we've gone off the proverbial deep end. Friends and family may object if we minister to society's outcasts such as prisoners and AIDS victims. "Aren't you going overboard with this religion thing?" they may ask. "Church on Sunday is fine, but why are you doing this other stuff?" But have courage! Jesus himself encountered resistance: "When his relations heard of this, they set out to take charge of him: they said, 'He is out of his mind'" (Mk 3:21).

Union with Christ means staying in ministry for the long haul rather than serving God for a short time and then saying, "Well, that was great. Now I need to do some other things." For over twenty years, a group of caring people in a Seattle parish have devoted themselves to serving dinner to the needy every Sunday. They treat their disheveled customers as though they were serving Christ himself. A few clients fight, show up drunk and harass people in the church where the dinner is held. This, in turn, leads some people to complain about the fiscal and emotional costs to the parish, but the dinners endure.

If we become holy, we, too, can expect the disapproval of those who fail to understand what it means to live in union with Christ, year-in and year-out. But our quiet endurance will model Christ in Christian communities that all too often surrender to the malady of apathy. James called this faith without works and questioned it harshly:

> How does it help, my brothers, when someone who has never done a single good act claims to have faith? Will that faith bring salvation? If one of the brothers or one of the sisters is in need of clothes and has not enough food to live on, and one of you says to them, "I wish you well, keep yourself warm and eat plenty," without giving them these bare necessities of life, then what good is that? In the same way faith: if good deeds do not go with it, it is quite dead (Jas 2:14–17).

Holiness eventually brings us face to face with evil. The sheer magnitude of its presence in today's world can overwhelm us when we compare it to our feeble goodness. Evil will win out, we say, because it's so huge and we're so small. Yet Jesus robbed Satan of his power over death when he died on the cross. Our baptism into the death and resurrection of Christ gives us the power to confront evil without being destroyed. With the psalmist we can say "I should fear no danger, for you are at my side" (Ps 23:4b).

Many people experience evil in the form of indirect opposition to ministry — a sick child prevents them from keeping an appointment for ministry, an argument with a friend distracts a minister from focusing well during prayer. We who minister religious healing need not crumble in the face of this reality. Instead, we should pray for protection from evil on behalf of ourselves and our loved ones. This will diminish much of its power — but not all of it. The more we serve Christ, the more we threaten the kingdom of darkness. Evil will oppose our ministry in the hopes of getting us to quit. At the Last Supper Jesus warned us of what comes with the job description of being his servant:

> Remember the words I said to you: A servant is not greater than his master. If they persecuted me, they will persecute you too (Jn 15:20a).

The Privilege of Mission

As we stare at the costs of ministry, we naturally might conclude that only a lunatic would sign up for this kind of program. But ministry is a two-sided coin, with one side being cost and the other privilege. In saying "yes" to God, we will experience not just the challenge of mission, but also its *privilege*.

Before his ascension, Jesus said to his disciples:

> All authority in heaven and on earth has been given to me. Go, therefore, make disciples of all nations. And look, I am with you always; yes, to the end of time (Mt 28:18b, 19a, 20b).

What a blessing to have our Lord and savior with us always and in every circumstance! What an honor to share in fulfilling the Father's dream for creation! Could any value exceed being the hands, feet, eyes — the very Body — of Christ in today's world? Our dignity as sons and daughters of God defies description.

On a down-to-earth level, we experience the privilege of ministry as we join people during a profound phase of their journey with God. Sharing with those who are at a difficult time in their lives is like assisting at a birth — the birth of new life that will endure for all eternity, the birth of a child of God into more and more of God's fullness. These are sacred moments, and the blessing is as much ours as it is theirs because, through ministry, we ourselves experience God's love in a very specific and particular way. Ministry helps us grow in our knowledge of the Lord; we come to know God on a more intimate level.

When we look at all the costs and privileges of ministry, we might share Isaiah's feelings at the time of his call: "Woe is me! I am lost, for I am a man of unclean lips and I live among a people of unclean lips, and my eyes have seen the King, Yahweh Sabaoth" (Is 6:5). But God asks us to unite ourselves with him in a sacred task — in spite of our weaknesses, in spite of the sacrifices, in spite of our feelings of unworthiness. He says, "Whom shall I send? Who will go for us?" and asks us to say, with Isaiah, "Here am I, send me" (Is 6:9).

Summary

A. The church is a community with the mission of carrying on the task given to Jesus by the Father: to bring forth the kingdom of God. Christians are first called then sent forth to minister God's healing love to a wounded world. Some of them are commissioned by the church as qualified for a specific healing ministry, while others engage in non-commissioned ministry of reaching out to hurting people in the name of Jesus.

B. Ministry has two costs:

1. The sacrifice of time and energy, including taking the time to get trained for ministry. Spiritual formation is crucial because effective ministers must have "the mind of Christ" (1 Cor 2:16b).

2. The price of holiness, which includes experiencing our spiritual poverty, the disapproval of others, the reality of evil, and the pain of compassion.

C. Ministry is also a privilege:

1. God is with us at all times.

2. We join people during a phase of their journey with God.

3. We share in fulfilling God's dream for creation.

Chapter Five

The Power of Community

*Why are prayer teams a powerful source of
healing wounds, and how do teams function?*

Community has the power to wound, community has the power to heal. Consider, for example, the power the community can exert after a premature birth. When communities use their power as God intends, the tiny baby is welcomed with loving concern by medical staff, parents, relatives, neighbors, friends, and the church. In the neonatal unit, doctors and nurses devote weeks to monitoring her condition. The pastor comes to the hospital shortly after delivery and baptizes the child. The parish prays for the baby by putting her on a "prayer chain." Grandparents visit the hospital to see the baby and offer support to the anxious parents. A far away relative sends a book on "preemies" and their care. Friends who also have gone through the experience of having a premature baby phone to say, "We know how difficult this time is for you."

As the time approaches to take the child home, relatives host baby showers, where the baby receives "adorable" clothing, etc. During the first exhausting days at home, parishioners drop off dinners. When the mother has trouble with nursing, the La Leche League provides help. With the parents' blessing, pastoral visitors come to the home several times to pray for the family and for the baby's recovery from her newborn experiences of isolation, pain and physical danger.

The above situation demonstrates the community's power to heal. First the baby's life is saved, then she experiences healing from her traumatic beginnings. The parents feel loved and supported by a number of communities — medical, parish, geographic, and family.

But communities do not always use their power in the way God intends. Instead of healing, sometimes they wound. Take another case, that of a pregnant high school student. Parents of the unwed mother respond with horror to news of her pregnancy. "What will the family say?" her father shouts. They threaten to kick her out of their home but then relent. Thus begin day-in and day-out put-downs: "We *told* you not to go out with that guy. Why don't you ever listen to us?"

By the grace of God, the teenager endures her family's condemnation, but her school community finishes the job of destroying her. The school counselor and classmates badger her to get an abortion. When she resists their coercion, one student after another tells her she's being "dumb." However, their real condemnation begins when she reveals she's going to put the baby up for adoption. "How can you give your baby away?" they say. "Don't you love it?"

Ultimately her family encounters the public shame they feared. Neighbors, church members, relatives all gossip behind the family's back. A few criticize them to their faces. The parents respond to their growing isolation by making their daughter's life a living hell. Crushed by her church, school and family communities, finally she runs away.

Community: A Life-or-Death Need

Few people perceive the immense power the community wields for better or for worse in every individual's life. Even when recognizing their power to hurt or to heal, many communities fail to take responsibility for this power. Some experts say it's due to apathy. Psychiatrist M. Scott Peck says it's caused by laziness and calls it the opposite of love:

> When we extend ourselves, when we take an extra step or walk an extra mile, we do so in opposition to the inertia of laziness or the resistance of fear. . . . Love is a form of work or a form of courage. Specifically, it is work or courage directed toward the nurture of our own or another's spiritual growth. . . . If an act is not one of work or courage, then it is not an act of love. There are no exceptions.[1]

In the case of the previously mentioned preemie baby, the communities surrounding the family worked hard and courageously to support them in a time of crisis. They acted with love, and the power of that love healed parents and baby.

In the case of the pregnant teenager, no community responded with love. In a fit of laziness or fear, no one was willing to walk an extra mile with a hurting, unmarried mother. Everyone used the power of their community to wound instead of heal, to hurt instead of love.

Humans cannot be fully human without membership in some organized group. This is the source of the power that communities wield over us. We Americans have trouble recognizing this power because our society is so pluralistic. If we're rejected by one community — or if we reject it ourselves — we can turn to another.

At certain stages, such as infancy and old age, we cannot even survive outside a community. Jan once gave physical therapy treatments to an elderly man who had been abandoned in a house by his caregivers. By the time someone found him, he was near death from dehydration and starvation. He had been sitting in a wheelchair during his whole ordeal, so his hip and knee joints were nearly fused into that position. It took many painful months of care and treatment to correct the damage caused by a one-week absence of a community.

Even the strong and robust need community just to gain a sense of being alive. Teenagers demonstrate this every day by their relentless search for a group — *any* group — with which they can identify. If they don't find a positive one in sports, parish, music, school, etc., they locate a harmful one in street gangs, drug subcultures, etc. When teens are asked why they join a gang when they know they might die as a result, they frequently say, "Well, at least in a gang I'm *somebody*." Exactly. Without a community, we are a bunch of nobodies, lacking what only a group can give.

Community: Giver of World Views

Communities give individuals their world view, a sense of how the world "works." This includes moral values, religious ideas, ideas about health and sickness, attitudes about relationships, and perspectives about the environment. A child who grows up seeing his father as the authority figure in the home will think that's how families work. A Hindu who believes cows are sacred will gaze with horror upon a Christian who eats beef. A logger who thinks that forests

contain an endless supply of wood will clash with an environmental-
ist who figures that no such eternal supply exists.

Few people question the world views held by their community.
They conform. To do otherwise creates the risk of ostracism, which
threatens their existence. The logger who becomes an environmen-
talist risks getting fired and being unable to support his family. The
boy who grows up and becomes a house-husband faces ridicule from
other men and, perhaps, women.

Most people who reject their community's world view leave that
group and join one with a view that matches theirs. Adolescents
do this with distressing regularity, especially as regards their family and religious communities. The hippie movement in the 1960s
was a massive rebellion of youth against the values of their childhood
communities. They left those groups to form their own communities
of people who shared their ideals. Some sank into a haze of drugs,
where the group "tuned out" to everyone except themselves. Others, however, created the civil rights and peace movements where,
united, they confronted the opposing world view of "the system."

Occasionally a genius, a charismatic figure or a select group
comes along who can change a portion of the world view of a given
community while still remaining within it. For instance, Pope John
XXIII came to the papacy at a time when the church considered itself the "perfect society" and saw the world as dangerous.[2] Until the
1960s, Catholics rallied around themselves to form a bulwark against
godless values. In only a few years' time, Pope John XXIII managed
to change this bastion mentality. He called Catholics to transform
the world, not shun it. The attitude of a perfect, hierarchal society
receded and was replaced by the people of God — real, collegial,
in love with all of God's creation, and committed to caring for it. In
less than a decade, Pope John XXIII altered the world view of the
Catholic church.

Those who strive to change a group from within pay a price for
doing so. At the very least, they are lonely in the midst of those they
care about. At worst, they are killed. Martin Luther King, Jr. devoted
his life to changing America's attitudes toward African-Americans
and their place in our society. We remember the successes of his
final days, just as we remember the triumph of Pope John XXIII's efforts. But King spent months in jail, suffered frequent rejection from
whites and ultimately was assassinated. He paid dearly for changing
America's views.

Sometimes a change of world view is for good; sometimes it is for ill. A teenager who rejects Christianity and moves into a live-for-the-thrills life of violence is not moving forward. A society that adopts a looking-out-for-number-one attitude is not improving itself. In the U.S., the value of communal responsibility has gradually evolved into the supremacy of the individual. The so-called "right to privacy" now legally supercedes the right to life. Individual freedom of expression includes the right to publish hate literature against groups a person dislikes. Where communities used to form strong bonds for nurturing and support, they now form loose-knit connections to be used, service stations for refueling. This change of world view from relationships to individualism is impacting our lives and attitudes as Christians.

The Body of Christ as Community

The Body of Christ is a faith community, not just a belief system. Real people with real names gather together in real buildings to worship, strengthen and sustain each other. As with any community, the Body of Christ possesses its own world views, some good and some bad. We flinch at the anti-Semitism that has afflicted Christianity almost since its inception, while at the same time we rejoice in the church's proclamation of love for all humanity. Darkness and light co-exist within any community, and the Body of Christ is no exception.

How can a community which is an extension of Christ's presence on earth possess distorted world views? If the Body of Christ is of divine origin, why has it so often misread God's will during the course of its history? In religious healing, why do Christians differ so strongly in their ideas of what constitutes good ministry? The church has struggled with these questions for decades without reaching any clear-cut conclusions. Sin and redemption remain a mystery, and people who belong to — or want to belong to — the Body of Christ face a package deal: accept the imperfect with the perfect, or be resigned to a life of isolation or conflict. Most choose the first course of action, yielding to an influence which brings them love, growth and redemption, and sometimes prejudice, rigidity, and woundedness.[3]

Christianity's past overflows with examples of the Body of Christ wounding people, and we ministers of religious healing should expect to encounter these people often in our ministry. One frequent wound is a distorted image of God. Some Catholics carry with them a vision of "God the Checker," tallying up sins in a divine supermarket. He charges precise amounts for each sin: this much for missing mass on Sunday, that much for swearing, that much for yelling at the kids. Finally, the reckoning comes: x years in purgatory; no going to hell because the shopper cashes in some "coupons" of good deeds: one for helping an elderly neighbor, another for contributing to a food bank, etc.

Wounded Protestants rarely possess a supermarket image of God. If their community has implanted a view of a judgmental God within them, it usually revolves around one question: Are they *really* saved? For instance, a woman has dedicated her life to ministry in her church, yet she is tormented about her salvation. "Did I *really* give my life to Christ when I was sixteen," she asks, "or did I just say the words? Was I truly sincere?" The question haunts her.

Many sources for healing exist within the Body of Christ. The sacraments are some of the most potent ones. Another is the prayer team, sometimes called a healing team. The rest of this chapter focuses on prayer teams, first giving an overview of them and then discussing the remarkable power they possess.

The Prayer Team: An Overview

A prayer team consists of two, three, or four people who function as a unit ministering religious healing. Most teams are comprised of lay people only, but some have women religious as members, and a few include ordained clergy. Ideally, both genders are represented on a team because each possesses unique gifts. Since God contains the depths of both the masculine and the feminine, we need both genders to fully represent the traits of God. Unfortunately, most prayer teams function without men because more women than men engage in healing ministry.

Every team member has been given gifts by the Holy Spirit, and the combination of these gifts exceeds the sum of the individual ones. Herein lies a source of great power. Every team, with its mixture of talents, personalities and special gifts, makes Christ present to a supplicant more effectively than any one member could do alone.

To reach their fullest power, prayer teams need to feel called by God to this ministry, as individuals *and* as a team. This gives them an awareness of belonging. Without this sense of "rightness," ministers consume spiritual and emotional energy wondering if God is or is not calling them to this ministry. For instance, Leo spent the first few years of his priesthood wrestling with doubts about his preaching. Intellectually he knew God had called him to proclaim the good news to people, but he didn't *feel* called. Finally, a sense of "rightness" about his ministry came to him. From then on, his shortcomings in the pulpit became a challenge instead of an embarrassment. His awareness of being in the right place freed up his energies to focus on ministry, not on himself.

The most effective prayer teams have their call to ministry confirmed by some ecclesiastical authority to whom they are accountable. Accountability is vital for the success of healing ministry (including parish-based ministry), but confidentiality must be maintained. Ideally, teams hold regular meetings with an ordained or appointed leader so that he or she can give feedback on the ministry. They can discuss the ministry in general but must not discuss the names or details of any supplicant's problems. Accountability to an official or semi-official denominational body (e.g., a parish or a denominational prayer meeting) lends support to the team. Also, it safeguards teams from the sort of self-deception that destroyed Lila's ministry (in Chapter 2).

The most effective teams work as a unit for an extended time period, although some consist of strangers who come together on a spur-of-the-moment basis at, say, a religious convention. The latter pray in response to Jesus' promise that where two or more gather in his name, he is present. This is true, but impromptu prayer teams rarely function with great power because they are not yet *fully* gathered and united with one another in Christ's name. Members do not know each other's personalities, talents and charisms. Because they are strangers, or near strangers, they cannot draw courage and support from each other. Casual prayer teams are like any casual acquaintances. They tend not to get into depth because they aren't bonded to one another.

Teams minister to supplicants who request prayer for physical, emotional, spiritual or relational problems. A session may last for about one hour, and normally a team meets with a supplicant for a number of times, say six to eight times. This extended time period is important because healing is a journey, not a one time treatment. Accompanying supplicants on a journey towards wholeness increases the likelihood that their healings will last for all eternity, rather than fade like a dream at daybreak.

During ministry sessions, one person functions as the leader and the rest as team members. Team members support the leader, while the leader's main job is to coordinate the exercise of the gifts that the Holy Spirit has given to each member. Other, less vital, leadership tasks are keeping track of time, being the spokesperson for the team, and welcoming the supplicant; these tasks may be delegated to other team members; the coordinating of the gifts cannot. The team's respect and support for one another creates a unity that possesses great power. A dynamic flows from members to leader, from leader to members, and amongst the entire team, including the supplicant. Bonds of love grow from this respect. This is the love that heals.[4]

A team's ultimate source of unity lies in each person's relationship with Jesus, which has been nurtured and developed within their individual faith communities. Members need not be of the same denomination, but the world view of their respective communities must be similar enough so that they can function in a united way. For instance, if someone has been taught that psychology and medicine are evil, while someone else has learned to see them as healing gifts from God, these people will make poor teammates.

One final point must be made in this overview of prayer teams: *a team's primary task is to make God real to the supplicant.* The first step to achieving this goal is to establish a relationship with the supplicant, one that is characterized by warmth, empathy and sincerity. Then the prayer team creates a worship experience for the supplicant that is tailor-made for her needs.

The Power of a Prayer Team

The power of a prayer team stems from its being a small Christian community — a cell in the Body of Christ — with all the impact that communities make in people's lives. It is a community that knows its power and has consciously decided to use it to heal others. It invites people into its midst for awhile so that they can get well.

Prayer teams possess one underlying power that heals people: *the power of love.* When a small community devotes its energies to caring for the needs of an individual, asking for *nothing* in return — no fee, no required membership in their organization, no exploitation of the person's vulnerability — the experience heals. Few ever receive the blessing of a community's giving them their undivided attention over a period of months. Few ever are accepted unconditionally, even in our Christian culture. But when a community does love someone in this fashion, he is transformed.

If prayer teams possess so much power, why isn't team ministry present in every parish in the world? If these small communities can heal in such profound ways, why aren't healings common? We believe the scarcity of prayer teams and the rarity of healings are due to the fact that love is a burden. Yet if we are willing to accept that burden, healing will occur. To facilitate that we have identified five aspects of the love we are called to share. We call each aspect of love a power, because it is in these aspects we discover the healing power of love.

The power of hospitality

Say the word "hospitality" and most people picture someone offering them hors d'oeuvres on a tray. American society uses the word as the rough equivalent of politeness and good manners. Our Judeo-Christian heritage, however, equates hospitality with life itself. The desert communities of our ancestors recognized it as essential for survival. Therefore, in both the Hebrew and Christian scriptures, hospitality is a sacred duty (cf. Dt 10:18–19, 1 Pet 4:9). Jesus even said that our willingness to be hospitable will impact us on Judgment Day ("... I was a stranger and you made me welcome.... " Mt 25:33ff). When St. Paul exhorted early Christians to "look for opportunities to be hospitable" (Rom 12:13), he spoke from his ancient Jewish tradition.

The Hebrew scriptures record that any traveling stranger was entitled to hospitality from any host, even from his enemy. Specific rules of etiquette applied for both host and stranger. The host's duty was to do his best to transform the stranger into an honored guest and then send him forth to continue his journey in a restored state (cf. Gn 18:1ff). Having accepted a stranger into his home or community, the host now became bound to protect him from any danger, even at the cost of his own life or the life of loved ones (cf. Gn 19:2–8). The stranger, on the other hand, was prohibited from insulting the host or usurping his role. He was supposed to accept what was offered him and limit his stay to no longer than three days.

The need for hospitality is no less pressing today, although current needs often center more around emotions and spirituality rather than food, shelter and water. We still travel in a desert, in the aridity of life's journey. Because we are relational creatures, our spiritual and emotional survival depends upon the willingness of others to offer us hospitality. At certain moments we cannot make it without the help of others. It's at these times that God asks Christians to take strangers into their *hearts*, to love them and heal them so that they can go forth, restored, to continue their journey through life.

Unfortunately, the church's ministry to hurting people often features professionalism without hospitality. Ministry occurs at arms' length, where the minister feels good about helping people without having plunged into the risk of loving them. Knowledge and skill are essential, but without love, ministers are "a gong booming or a cymbal clashing." Worse yet, without love ministers are "nothing" (1 Cor 13:1–2).

The power of hospitality is the power of love. If prayer teams offer a supplicant nothing more than their hospitality, this act itself is healing. By welcoming a hurting person into their hearts, team members remove isolation, helplessness and hopelessness — three major blocks to healing (Chapter 9 expands on this topic). A supplicant who experiences the unconditional love of a prayer team is free to be herself, with no mask and no role to play. She can safely try out new behavior without being committed to it and without fear of the criticism she might encounter with, say, her family.

The potency of hospitality's love makes it likely that a supplicant will do almost anything to keep on receiving it. This can be a positive force for enabling her to overcome the fear and inertia that often blocks healing. Yet a team can use hospitality as a negative force by exploiting the supplicant's need for community. Cults are prime examples of the misuse of the power of hospitality. After inviting vulnerable people into their midst and appearing to love them unconditionally, they systematically rob them of their freedom by physically, mentally and spiritually controlling them for the cult's benefit.

Few prayer teams misuse the power of hospitality with the intensity of a cult. But they can succumb to a more subtle version of control by making their love *conditional*. Instead of extending Jesus' unqualified love, some teams pull back emotionally when a supplicant doesn't do what they want. For instance, if a Catholic supplicant decides to get married outside the church, the team may give off an emotional chill that was not present earlier. This experience can add one more wound to an already wounded life and will distract the supplicant from her primary goal in life, namely, to become the person God wants her to be. Without unconditional love, team ministry can be more hurtful than helpful.

The greatest gift of hospitality is the freedom it offers the supplicant. God calls us to love others without taking away their freedom, but this is extraordinarily difficult. In the presence of someone's pain, our conviction that Jesus is Lord tends to vanish and be replaced by the idea that God expects us to be saviors. Sociologist Parker Palmer calls this aberration "salvation by interaction" and believes the church is riddled with an obsession to fix other people's problems:

> This is a hidden doctrine of salvation that runs through a lot of our church life; and ironically it pushes us apart from each other because you don't want the burden of trying to save me, which you can't do anyway. And I sure don't want the burden of you trying to save me.
>
> What people need to be able to do is to sit and listen to another person's deepest concerns with a real confidence that salvation doesn't come from us, to be confident that this language about God moving in our lives to heal and transform others is not just blowing smoke. To sit in that way is to sit in a very different relation to our problems.[5]

The most common abuse of hospitality, however, is its absence. Prayer teams expend great physical, emotional and spiritual energy when they welcome a hurting person into their hearts. Sharing someone's pain takes stamina. Why put ourselves out for a woman on a journey of transformation? Why go out on a rainy night to listen to a man's anguish? The answer is that Jesus asks us to "go out to the whole world; proclaim the gospel to all creation" (Mk 16:15). When we respond to this command, mysteriously we find ourselves blessed. Those who welcome strangers into their hearts invariably report they have received more than they've given. Hospitality blesses us more than it blesses the stranger.

The power of pastoral listening

Few wayfarers need a platter of food from us, but everyone has a need to be truly heard. Listening is the tool that hosts — and teams — use to access the power of hospitality. Imagine a host who never listens to a word his guest says. How can people welcome someone into their hearts if they never truly listen to him? How can a team know God's will for a supplicant if they fail to listen to her expressed needs?

These may appear to be obvious points, but many Christians are wretched listeners. They listen superficially to a supplicant's statement of a problem, and then assume they know what's going on. This deficiency robs their ministry of power and causes many of the pitfalls of ministry that we discuss in Chapter 7. True pastoral listening requires selflessness. For example, it requires that we give up the lure of "salvation by interaction" (the desire to rush in and "fix" someone's problem).

Chapter 6 shows how to use pastoral listening in healing ministry. Here we will note that listening possesses a power that goes beyond human action. It is a divine activity. Members of the Body of Christ make themselves fully present to people in faith, out of love and with hope. This leads supplicants to feel they have been heard not just by a team, but by God. They have an experience of a *listening* God who truly knows their need and is with them in that need. This alone is healing.

The power of expectations

We believe that expectations play such a powerful role in healing that we've devoted an entire chapter to the subject (Chapter 10). Few people are healed without first *expecting* that something will happen to them, and usually that expectation must come from sources outside themselves. In the medical field it often comes from physicians and other caregivers. In religious healing it needs to come from the ministers.

The power of expectations arises from the individual's life-and-death need to be accepted by a community. Psychological studies reveal that people rise, or sink, to the level of expectation that a community has for them. For instance, when a teacher is told that a slow student is bright, his grades rise even if she never verbalizes her expectations to him. A prayer team that believes a supplicant will be healed greatly enhances the likelihood of that happening.[6]

Because a prayer team is a cell in the Body of Christ, supplicants usually see the team's expectations as carrying the authority of God. They start looking at themselves, God, events, illness, etc. the way the team does. This fact highlights the critical importance for a team's world view to conform with Christ's. St. Paul tells us to "put on the mind of Christ," and nowhere is that more critical than in seeing God's expectations for each individual who needs healing.

Teams that discern and express God's expectations for a particular supplicant in a particular ministry session transmit a powerful force for healing. (Chapters 9 and 10 explore this in depth.) A supplicant begins to *expect* that something good will happen and therefore opens himself up to that goodness.

Great harm can arise when the power of expectations is misused. For instance, if a team silently concludes that nothing is going to happen, usually nothing does. On the other hand, large healing services can manipulate people into "claiming" healings on the spot before any medical confirmation of those healings can occur. The leader of a service may announce that "right now the Lord is healing a woman's breast cancer," and someone will stand up and say that she's the person who's been healed. The leader's expectation has unintentionally pressed upon her a message that may not be true. If the woman later discovers that she hasn't been healed, a variety of destructive emotions will usually assail her: defeat, depression, distrust of healing ministry and false guilt. ("I didn't have enough faith to be healed.")[7]

The inevitable transferring of expectations from team to supplicant means that teams should know what those expectations are — both conscious and unconscious. This is not easy! It requires prayer, openness among team members, reflection on ministry and, sometimes, consultation with outside experts who can maintain the team's promise to the supplicant of confidentiality. Knowing what it expects helps a team reject those expectations that do not reflect God's will and embrace those that do. A team that identifies God's specific desires for each supplicant is a team with a powerful ministry.

The power of role models

In some ways, role modeling in ministry resembles role modeling in parenting. A child admires his parents' power and very existence, so he tries to be like them. His life-or-death need for approval from his community (i.e., the parents) makes role modeling a key force in his life. What mom and dad *say* is not nearly so important as who mom and dad *are*. If they nurture their child, he will tend to become a nurturer; if they see God as a loving parent, he probably will develop the same vision.

For better or for worse, those of us who minister healing prayer are role models. Supplicants come for prayer and end up seeing reality as we see it. They pick up our attitudes toward God, themselves and others. Usually this is a conscious process. They experience our helpfulness and compassion and decide that they, too, would like to be helpful and compassionate. Our prayer in ministry inspires them to enter into deeper prayer in their everyday life.

For instance, our friends Dave and Iris Beardemphl periodically give a one-day seminar entitled "The Family That Prays Together, Stays Together." After each seminar, a few couples decide to use Dave and Iris' explicit prayer examples in their own families, e.g., the father begins to bless his children in the same way that Dave has described his blessing of his children and grandchildren. Months after a seminar, a woman will come up to Iris and say, "We've been doing just what you and Dave do, and it works! Our family life has completely turned around."

What holds true for the positive side of role modeling also holds true for the negative. If we see God as vengeful and poised to destroy us, a supplicant might adopt the same attitude. Even positive modeling can become negative if it clashes with the world view of a supplicant's faith community. For instance, a Catholic prayer team that introduces a Presbyterian supplicant to the use of sacramentals may cause more harm than good if her family and congregation believe that sacramentals are evil. Rejection by a community creates new pain and slows healing, so in prayer ministry we must exercise caution in how we model God, faith and ourselves to our supplicants. Our role modeling may not exactly match their community's world view, but it shouldn't oppose it.

The burden of role modeling is that sometimes we'd like to plug in the message of "don't do as I *do*, just do as I *say*." Actually, that expression doesn't communicate the power — and burden — of role modeling. Really, we'd like to say "don't be as I am," because sometimes we aren't what we'd like to be. The thought of someone embodying all that we are — for better *and* for worse — is a chilling idea. We would prefer that supplicants pick up the positive from us and let the negative slip quietly into the night.

Supplicants can separate our positive traits from our negative ones if their imitation of us is a conscious choice, as it has been with Dave and Iris' seminar. But deeply wounded supplicants tend to copy us unconsciously, almost as if they want to be our clones.

These people have less ability to separate the negative from the positive. Either way, whether we're dealing with a conscious or unconscious process, ministers of religious healing are powerful models for those we serve. Therefore, we need to continually strive for maturity, growth, and virtue.

The power of being Christ-bearers

Being a Christ-bearer is one of the little-known powers of healing ministry. A supplicant sees a team and its members as being more than just themselves. In her eyes, we healing ministers are larger than life because we symbolize the church, the Christian community and even God. We think of ourselves as normal people who put our pants on one leg at a time, but a supplicant may view us as being one step below divine. If so, she will attribute huge importance to our every word and action.

Leo recalls an incident when he was fresh out of the seminary and assigned to do six weeks of hospital ministry. There he met a twentieth-century version of the woman at the well (Jn 4:4–42). The patient had had multiple husbands, was alienated from God and church, and had committed a stunning array of sins over a twenty-five year period. An automobile accident put her in the hospital, where Leo found her suspended in traction and swathed in bandages from head to toe. Feeling inadequate about his pastoral care abilities, Leo listened to the woman for awhile, then said a ritual blessing. Looking at her immobilized state and not knowing what else to say, he cracked a joke as he left: "Well, don't do anything I wouldn't do!"

Leo visited the woman two days later and was astounded to hear her say that she'd been thinking about his parting statement ever since. "I've been comparing what I've done with what you do as a priest," she said, "and I've decided I've made a mess of my life. I want to change." Thereupon she said she wanted to make a general confession. Leo was flabbergasted that someone could take a flippant statement and turn it into a source of conversion. What he didn't realize until years later was that, in the eyes of this patient, he was a bearer of Christ, a living sacrament who momentarily was God to her.

Christ-bearers are a part of a supplicant's world view of God and community. This can work for ministry or against it, depending on what the team symbolizes to the supplicant. For instance, a man who believes that people are hyper-critical often will see the team in the same way. Like a circus mirror that makes even thin people look fat, to him all ministry will feel laden with criticism and condemnation. On the other hand, a woman who sees people as supportive will view the team in the same fashion. This will enhance ministry because she will find it relatively easy to trust the team and allow them to minister God's love to her.

We must get used to the fact that supplicants place more importance in our words and actions than we intend. We cannot dissuade them from doing so and therefore should resist the urge to say, "Quit genuflecting to us!" We may cringe when someone sees us as being an image of God or of church instead of just ourselves. But being Christ-bearers is a power that can link us to a supplicant's mind and emotions and create a channel through which God can heal.

Conclusion

All of the powers a prayer team possesses come from God through the natural and supernatural gifts he bestows on us. Even with these gifts, however, we need empowerment by the Holy Spirit every time we minister. Ministry is like a sailboat that needs wind each time it sets sail. It cannot go anywhere on the basis of past, glorious experiences. Jesus said, "By myself I can do nothing" (Jn 5:30a), and the same holds true for us. To be effective, our ministry must be grounded in radical dependency on God's power. The breath of the Holy Spirit must fill every moment of the work we do in the name of the Lord. This requires great humility!

To serve the Lord effectively, we must rid ourselves of the illusion of self-power and face the fact that, like Jesus, alone we can do nothing. With God, however, and within the community of a prayer team, powers come to us that we otherwise do not possess. When we use these powers for good, we become channels for God's healing love. Love is a responsibility, but love unites us with the one who raised Jesus from the dead, the one who now asks us to help complete Christ's task of recreating the universe.

Summary

Community has the power to heal and to wound because people are relational beings who need community for their very survival. The community gives world views to its members, a sense of how the world "works." These views include moral values, religious ideas plus attitudes toward health and sickness.

The Body of Christ is a community that possesses its own world views, some good and some bad. Prayer teams are a powerful source of healing for wounded members of a faith community.

A prayer team consists of two, three, or four people who feel called by God to minister as individuals and as a team. Ideally, their call is confirmed by some ecclesiastical authority to whom they are accountable and to whom they make a commitment to work as a unit for an extended time period. Teams minister to supplicants who request prayer for physical, emotional, spiritual or relational problems. *Their primary task is to make God real to the supplicant.*

Prayer teams possess one underlying power that heals people: the power of love. That is communicated in five different ways:

1. the power of hospitality;
2. the power of pastoral listening;
3. the power of expectations;
4. the power of role modeling;
5. the power of being Christ-bearers.

All of a prayer team's power must be activated by the Holy Spirit each time it ministers.

Chapter Six

Healing Ministry Is Worship

*Why does religious healing fall into the category
of worship, and how can ministers create a
worship experience for someone who is hurting?*

Anthony Andrews was in the grip of pain, but he wasn't alone. His whole family was caught in the same grip with him. He had just been told that he had bone cancer. In distress, the Andrews turned to a member of their parish and asked for help. She, in turn, asked Leo for assistance.

When he met with the Andrews, Leo observed that Anthony was in pain and seemingly in shock, while his wife Estelle was overcome with emotion. Leo was concerned about Anthony's physical pain, as well as his emotional and spiritual suffering. But he saw that Anthony's family also had many emotional and spiritual needs.

The Andrews told Leo they wanted to deal with this illness as a family, so Leo suggested they receive ongoing prayer ministry plus the sacrament of anointing of the sick for Anthony. A week later three generations gathered to celebrate the anointing of the sick. Present were Leo, Anthony, Estelle, two children and three grandchildren. A parish prayer team joined them.

The session began with everyone placed in a circle. As Leo progressed through the rite of anointing, he described each step. After reading James 5:14, he explained that all present were more than spectators; they were active members of the Body of Christ. Therefore, healing would flow from them as well as from Leo. He then read a scripture passage about one of Jesus' healings and said he believed Jesus would do the most loving thing possible in this situation. He laid his hands on Anthony's head, then invited the others,

77

including the grandchildren, to do likewise. The grandchildren responded solemnly with curiosity and awe. Anthony had tears in his eyes, and Estelle was sobbing.

Next Leo anointed Anthony with oil blessed by a bishop, said the ritual words of the sacrament, then prayed spontaneously. When he finished praying, he invited others to do likewise if they so desired. With Estelle's permission, one of the prayer ministers anointed her with oil blessed by a priest for lay use[1] and prayed for God to give her the grace to care for Anthony *and* herself. At the end of the one-hour session, Anthony and Estelle said they felt blessed by God through the sacrament, through the other prayers and through the presence of their loved ones.

What we've just described is healing ministry as the church intends it to be. A careful look reveals a common thread running through it: the entire session was one of worship. In fact, if understood properly, *healing ministry is worship.*

Worship in its broadest sense enables a person or a community to come before God with a need and, in the midst of praise and thanksgiving, to experience God meeting them in that need in the most loving way possible.[2] As a result of this personal encounter with God, the worshiper is transformed in some way. This is not the purpose of scientific medicine, whose goal is to cure disease. But transformation is precisely the purpose of the ministry of religious healing.

Practiced as worship, healing ministry liberates us from performance pressure, avoids practicing medicine, and takes us beyond counseling or mere petitions. It focuses on God, unites us with the Body of Christ and fills us with praise and thanksgiving. But in the face of pain or illness, worship doesn't occur easily; our temptation in distressing circumstances is to become goal oriented, e.g., this knee needs curing, this marriage needs fixing. Objectives like this are not enough to transform us into the wholeness of God. We need worship that brings us into the presence of the one who heals.[3]

With this in mind, the rest of this chapter shows how to create a worship experience for a supplicant. Also, it discusses criteria to use to evaluate the success or failure of ministry.

How to Make Healing Ministry an Experience of Worship

1. Create a sacred space.

It takes planning to make healing ministry an experience of worship. First we need to create a sacred space into which we invite people. Banners, other forms of sacred art, blessed candles, a Bible, comfortable chairs — all these can combine to create a mood of holiness. A sacred space makes a non-verbal statement. It says, "This is holy ground; come join us."

For example, before meeting with the Andrews' family in the parish rectory, Leo and the prayer team (Donna and Sharon) chose a room that already contained sacred art and comfortable chairs. Leo added a Bible, a blessed candle, oil blessed by the bishop, and some holy water. Donna brought with her some flowers from her garden. With these items arranged, the room felt warm, inviting, and ready for worship.

2. Gather as the Body of Christ.

Every Sunday the Body of Christ gathers at masses and services throughout the world. We who pray in seclusion each day set aside a time each week to pray in communion with others. Our public prayer differs from our private prayer as a violin solo contrasts with a symphony. Both are beautiful; neither can replace the other. Community worship brings a dimension of power into our lives that private worship lacks. In song, in prayer, in eucharist, in ritual, in scripture, and in union with others, a meeting takes place between God and his people. The power of this meeting removes our isolation and rejuvenates us.

As with Sunday worship, healing prayer increases in power and potential when done within a faith community. Prayer teams gather in the name of the Lord to focus on a supplicant and her needs. We place this person, her needs and ourselves before God, who uses us and our gifts to bring his grace into that need. A common way to begin a gathering of the Lord's people is with music. When we sing, we breathe together and become one in word and in spirit. A simple song such as "Peace is Flowing Like a River" takes us from our isolated thoughts. This, in turn, makes us aware of the presence of those around us. Together with the psalmist, we join our voices to glorify God:

Sing a new song to Yahweh:
his praise in the assembly of the faithful!
Israel shall rejoice in its maker,
the children of Zion delight in their king (Ps 149:1–2).

3. Create an awareness of God's presence.

During the course of the Andrews' prayer session, everyone became aware that God was truly there. Jesus' parting words to his disciples came to life: "And look, I am with you always; yes, to the end of time" (Mt 28:20b). Prayer teams need to create this awareness of God's presence. This is a challenging task!

Some people begin the process of making God real by simply inviting the Lord into the room, e.g., "Lord, we ask you to enter this room. Come join us here in our circle and fill us with your love . . . ." Actually, God already *is* present. We need to pray to recognize that fact. Those who don't do this may end up praying to God as though he were perched on Mars, aloof and removed from people's pain. If ministers pray in a remote fashion, that's how supplicants will experience God. One of our jobs is be sure this doesn't happen. We must make God *real* to our supplicants so that they can experience his love and care in the midst of their pain.

Scripture can create a powerful awareness of God's presence. One appropriate passage comes from Matthew: "For where two or three meet in my name, I am there among them" (Mt 18:20). This verse is helpful at the beginning of a healing ministry session because it brings the promise of Jesus into a ministry session. Jesus is truly present! This awareness raises everyone's expectant faith.

4. Focus on the supplicant's need.

Having created an awareness of God's presence, the ministry now can focus on the specific needs of the supplicant. Here's where listening skills become crucial. A team that listens well can empathize with a supplicant and establish rapport within in a surprisingly short time. Some supplicants experience healing just because the team listens to them! In our fast-paced society, people come to us who have never been truly listened to in their lives. We offer a priceless gift when we give them our full, loving attention.

Christian and secular literature abound with excellent books on listening.[4] Here, we'll simply describe one of the fruits of listening, namely knowing what needs to happen in this particular ministry session with this particular supplicant. Many people call this knowledge "discernment." It is the combination of a gift from God plus developed personal skills that, together, form a sense of the direction a ministry session should take.

The closest we can come to describing discernment is to say it feels like an inner conviction, a sense that *this* is the need to be ministered to, this is the place to begin. People with the gift of discernment explain this conviction in various ways — an inner light turning on inside their mind, a mental flag starting to wave, an inner "ah-ha" feeling. However it's described, discernment gives us a strong, peaceful "this fits" experience of rightness in a particular ministry session with a particular supplicant.

In discernment, we place ourselves and our supplicants in God's hands. We learn to listen simultaneously to the Lord, to our team members, to our supplicant and to our inner selves. At first, it feels as though we need four brains and three sets of ears to exercise discernment, but in fact, good listening skills give us the ability to become like parents who sort through their children's cares and deal with the essential needs of the moment. Bombarded with laughing, crying, noisy, always needful children, parents discern from moment to moment when and how they need to respond. In ministry, we do likewise.

Prayer teams can be aided in their discernment process by starting with one question: What is the supplicant ready for at this time? This is not the same as asking what the most basic need is. Confusion between need and readiness leads to poor ministry and sometimes even disasters. For instance, someone may come to us asking for physical healing for low back pain, and we discern that the backache arises from stresses in relationships at home. If we ignore the request for prayer for physical healing and launch into prayer for relationships, we leap ahead of God, who always loves and accepts us *as we are* and moves forward with us from that point.

The hallmark of effective prayer ministry is that we, like Jesus, *accept people where they are and journey with them from there.* Good discernment starts with this realization. Prayer for any type of healing often leads supplicants into deeper issues. What starts as prayer for, say, an ailing shoulder, may lead to prayer for other issues. Once the door has been opened to God, wonders can happen. With this knowledge, we progress to the next step in making healing ministry an experience of worship.

5. Enter into the heart of worship.

This means pray, pray, pray! In healing ministry, the heart of worship is a liturgy tailor-made for this supplicant with this need at this moment — a prayer meeting for one person. It includes riches of prayer that have woven themselves through thousands of years of Judeo-Christianity.

In the heart of worship, we let God's grace flow *through* us. God is truly present within us and wants to use us as channels of his healing grace. As we allow him to do this, we suddenly know that the statement "only God heals" is not true. Ever since God took on a human nature 2,000 years ago, he has been calling us — and empowering us — to share in his work. We share in this mission when we become fully present to God and fully present to the supplicant. In deep worship, God's power flows through us. Healing occurs.

A common mistake in healing ministry is to restrict prayer to one form: petition (e.g., "Lord, heal Joe's back"). When religious healing is worship, however, we make use of many prayer forms, one of which is *praise and thanksgiving.* Follow-up ministry sessions with the Andrews by Donna and Sharon were filled with the wonder of Anthony and Estelle's marriage and of God's presence with them. They described their ministry sessions as "a place of praise." The Andrews' situation illustrates that when healing ministry is worship, praise spills out — praise for God's past and present blessings, for his presence in the current need, for the supplicant's inner beauty, etc. This brings God's power into ministry because, in the words of the psalmists, "The Lord inhabits the praises of his people."

Prophecy is a second form of prayer we can use in healing ministry. This is *not* foretelling the future. Rather, a team member feels inspired to speak to the supplicant with an "I" statement as though with God's voice. The prophecy brings hope and comfort to the supplicant because in a deep, personal way, it says, "I, the Lord, am with you. I love you."

Often prophecy takes the form of a scripture passage that applies directly to the needs of the supplicant. Hundreds of verses speak words of love and divine presence that supplicants may never have heard. This has a powerful impact because the word of God suddenly becomes *real* for this moment and this need. Donna and

Sharon used several scripture passages that Anthony and Estelle found comforting. They especially liked one from Isaiah:

> Do not be afraid, for I have redeemed you; I have called you by your name, you are mine. Should you pass through the waters, I shall be with you; or through rivers, they will not swallow you up. . . . For I am Yahweh, your God, the Holy One of Israel, your Savior (Is 43:1b–2a, 3a).

Prayer of affirmation is a nearly unknown prayer form that can transform someone's self-image. Here, ministers see a supplicant's positive traits and verbally pray to God in thanksgiving for those traits. In a prayer setting, people who normally ward off affirmation often accept a view of themselves that they would never before have dared to believe. Donna and Sharon always included prayers of affirmation in their ministry to the Andrews, e.g., "Thank you, Lord, for how Anthony loves and cherishes Estelle, for all the little ways he shows his love." Prayers of affirmation transform supplicants because they begin to see themselves as God sees them.[5]

Prayers of intercession certainly fall within the category of religious healing.[6] People come to us with hurts and we ask God to heal those hurts. But if intercession becomes the *only* form of prayer for healing, ministry degenerates into presenting a shopping list of requests to God. ("Oh Lord, heal Tom's wrist, find the right job for Wendy, protect the Smiths while they're traveling," etc.) This is not worship; it's a wish list mailed to a reluctant Santa secluded at the North Pole.

When intercession is a part of worship, we become so fully united with God, with the supplicant, with team members and with all of creation that a channel opens for God to work through us. The healing that follows comes from God as the source and from us, the team, as agents. Just as the vine needs branches for bearing fruit, and the branches need the vine for their very life, God and we work as one to bring about healing. In other words, healing flows through the Body of Christ.[7]

In Christ/we, incarnational intercessory prayer, God is not "out there" in space, waiting for us to dial the right spiritual number, find the right scripture promise, or say the right prayer. Instead, he is intimately present within us and within the supplicant, actually *eager* to do the most loving thing possible at this moment in time.

When the results of intercessory prayers disappoint us, we must face an unfortunate fact: What is wanted — by God, by us and by the supplicant — often is not possible. God has chosen to join us on earth. In so doing, he also has chosen to restrict himself in what he can do.

Sometimes God is restricted by the ministers. In Chapter 2, Lila failed in her discernment as well as in her sensitivity towards Henrietta. God would have had to violate all laws of love as well as reason in order to heal Henrietta through Lila's inept, over-powering ministry.

Sometimes God is restricted by a lack of readiness in the supplicant, even one who is growing. No one reaches God's wholeness instantly or completely, so a specific healing may not be feasible in a given situation at a given moment in time. For instance, a supplicant with emphysema may be growing in his relationship with God but nevertheless be unwilling to give up smoking. In that situation, our prayers for physical healing cannot counteract the damage caused by a continuing, three-pack-a-day habit. Our incarnational God does not remove the natural consequences of our behavior, no matter how fervently we pray.

Still other times, the environment holds God back from healing a supplicant. For example, an alcoholic who receives prayer for her compulsion to drink may lose her compulsion for alcohol — until she faces her family's continuing barrage of criticism, control, and assorted destructive behaviors. For her healing from addiction to be effective, her entire family would need relational healing, but they might balk at this. Or her ministers may lack the time, energy or knowledge of co-dependency to become channels of God's healing for this family at this time.

Discernment is crucial in intercessory prayer because it is linked to possibilities. As mentioned earlier, we must ask ourselves what is possible for this supplicant at this time. Even with good discernment, however, we often pray for one type of healing and another one occurs instead. A man seeking emotional healing discovers that first he needs spiritual healing. A woman asking for physical healing experiences a healing in her relationships. When encountering surprising results like these time and time again, we learn to bow to the mystery of God's action. We drop our demands for *this* result at *this* time in *this* ministry session and end up with one assurance: God always acts lovingly in good healing ministry.

A discussion of the different prayer forms we can use in worship could fill volumes, but a final one we'll touch on here is *praying with imagery*. Imagery is one of our most powerful tools for healing because no one can act beyond the images they hold about themselves and about others. Imagery determines our ability to act, think and feel because it is inseparable from thinking.[8] This fact forms the foundation of praying with imagery. When a supplicant's images change, she changes.

For example, Jan was once on a team that ministered to a woman we'll call Cecelia, who had suffered brutal abuse as a child. Her initial reason for seeking ministry was that she had a terror of God. The terror puzzled her because it did not fit with her feelings of love for God. After several sessions, the team discerned that, beneath her fear, Cecelia blamed God for her tragic childhood. They chose to use imagery to help her access this deep-seated feeling. The imagery prayer they selected was a scripture meditation: the passion of Christ.[9]

After briefly explaining scripture meditation to Cecelia, the team obtained her approval to use it to unearth the cause of her fear. Then while asking her to close her eyes and to place herself in the scripture scene, one team member began to slowly read the passion from Matthew's gospel. When the reader reached the verse describing Jesus' trial, Jan asked Cecelia where — and who — she was in the scene. "I'm one of people shouting "Crucify him!" she responded with a shudder. In that flash, she became aware of an anger she'd held within her for decades. She suddenly saw that her image of God was that of an all-powerful spectator who stood by for years while her father beat her and her mother criticized her relentlessly.

As Cecelia stayed with Jesus throughout his passion, her picture of him changed from his being powerful and aloof to his being vulnerable and loving. By the time she reached the foot of the cross, she realized that Jesus had suffered with her whenever she'd been beaten as a child. This awareness led to a turning point. Picturing herself standing at the foot of the cross, she experienced Jesus removing her heart of fear and anger and then replacing it with a heart of love.

We cannot think without using imagery, but these need not be visual. Researchers now believe that every person's mind operates through a "primary" sense, a key form of imagery through which he experiences reality. This sense may be visual, feeling, or auditory. When a prayer team uses imagery in healing ministry, it is helpful to discover what primary sense a supplicant uses because for imagery to be effective, the team must focus on that particular sense. In Cecelia's case, her primary sense of imagery was visual; she mentally *saw* herself in the gospel setting of Christ's passion. If her primary sense had been feeling, she would have had a *feeling* experience instead of a visual one. In either case, the use of imagery would emotionally involve her deeply.

Prayer teams need to discover what image of God is *safe* for their supplicant. A woman who has been the victim of rape may be terrified to envision an adult Jesus. Instead, she may prefer envisioning the infant Jesus with the holy family in Bethlehem. A few supplicants aren't comfortable with an image of Jesus in any form. One prayer team told us that, before entering into prayer with a supplicant, they ask: "When we say 'God,' what image comes to your mind?" Usually that's the person's safest one. They had one supplicant whose only safe image of God was the color green! After using this as the starting focus in prayer, she slowly shed her fears of God and grew in her ability to experience him in other safe ways.

Essentially, praying with images brings God into a supplicant's mind and allows her to think in new ways. Cecelia imaged herself being utterly alone as a child, and she imaged God being callously untouched by her abuse. Her anger about his inaction led her to see herself as being "bad." From this arose her fear of what would happen if she ever met God face-to-face. Prayer ministry changed Cecelia's image of aloneness to that of oneness with Christ. As her anger dissolved, so did her fear.

When using imagery for healing, external realities remain the same. What changes is *inner* reality — the way a person experiences those external facts. Cecelia's childhood abuse remained unchanged by ministry, but she became aware of God's presence in those moments. When she realized Jesus had suffered with her, her ways of thinking and feeling changed. She experienced a deep, spiritual healing and was released from the trap of her past abuse.

Imagery is a potent prayer form for all kinds of healing — emotional, spiritual, physical, and relational. Specific techniques vary according to the supplicant, the primary sense she uses and the type of healing needed. For instance, cancer patients often use imagery to picture chemotherapy drugs killing malignant cells; then they may image Jesus filling each cell in their body with light.[10] Regardless of the type of healing or the exact technique, this prayer form is a way to transform the meaning of a specific memory, emotion, relationship or health problem. Supplicants invite Jesus into themselves, *live* an experience with him, and know the truth as he knows it. In so doing, they are freed. Jesus' words come to life: "You will come to know the truth, and the truth will set you free" (Jn 8:32).

We end this section on worship by sounding a note of caution: Don't go beyond limitations! These fall into several categories. First, supplicants who are limited in their openness or in their exposure to some prayer forms will feel uncomfortable with certain kinds of prayer. Prophecy will puzzle someone who is unfamiliar with its proper usage. Praying with imagery might scare someone who is uncomfortable with an intimate God. So use *all* prayer forms with sensitivity.

Secondly, lack of time hampers our ability to do in-depth ministry with some supplicants. We must not open doors we cannot close! Cecelia's spiritual and emotional healing took place over a period of three months. If her awareness of her anger at God had come to her during, say, a large, one-time-only healing service, it would have devastated her. Having experienced her deep feelings, she needed strong support and several more ministry sessions to fully resolve her anger.

Another limitation exists in people's ability to handle what's revealed. Once the door to a person's heart, mind and soul opens, can the team and the supplicant handle what's behind the door? Sometimes the team can't handle it. For instance, a mature team that's knowledgeable about alcoholism will do better ministry to an alcoholic than will an unskilled team that has no information about the disease.

Sometimes supplicants cannot handle what's revealed in ministry. People can only bear so much growth within a given time period. We must respect each person's rate of growth. Forcing someone beyond his limits is like grabbing a rose bud and yanking its petals outward. It doesn't work. Worse yet, it destroys the rose.

6. *Bring worship to a close.*

In worship, the world outside the ministry room fades as everyone focuses on God's presence. This occurs in any powerful liturgy, whether it's a deeply moving mass or a powerful healing ministry session. To keep everyone from coming down with a case of spiritual "bends," we must end worship well.

As with any worship service, good closure includes expressing the fact that worship is coming to an end. Mass doesn't just quit, and neither should healing ministry. For example, mass doesn't end with people receiving communion and running out of church; so too, in healing ministry we must not end deep prayer one minute and shove the supplicant out the door the next!

Ending worship includes giving praise to God for the good he has done during the session. A period of praise seems to "seal" a healing that might otherwise be just a brief moment of relief in a lifetime of pain. Like a coating of varnish over a wood sculpture, praise puts the finishing touches on worship and healing. It increases the chances that a healing will last.

One ingredient of good closure is seeking feedback from the supplicant. What was helpful? What was unhelpful? Feedback clears up questions or misconceptions that either we or the supplicant may have. Without it, all sorts of assumptions can creep into minds and ministry. For instance, Lila felt no need to seek feedback in ministry. She assumed Henrietta's highly charged behavior arose from effective deliverance. Lila's first accurate feedback occurred when she heard she might be sued for emotional damages.

Before sending forth supplicants into the world, we need to help them plan for the future. If we will we do more ministry with them, it needs to be scheduled. If no further sessions are planned, do they need a referral to someone else for follow-up care? The "someone else" may be another prayer team, a physician or a psychologist. Follow-up also can include our encouragement for care that's already occurring outside of our ministry.

Bringing worship to a close always involves saying good-bye. Supplicants need to know we will not forget them. They need our assurance that we will keep them in our prayers. Some prayer teams demonstrate this assurance by giving their supplicants a token to take with them, e.g., a holy card or a scripture verse written down at the end of ministry. A brief prayer for God's protection is an especially comforting way to send forth supplicants into the world. Finally, if a person is open to it, good-bye hugs demonstrate our feelings for the supplicant and for what has occurred during ministry.

Criteria for Success/Failure in Ministry

If a man comes to us with a torn knee cartilage and his knee is cured during the course of our prayers, has our ministry been a success? Not necessarily. If his knee *isn't* cured, has our ministry been a failure? Not necessarily.

If we ask these questions in a medical setting the answers are obvious. But since we ministers of healing are not practicing medicine, our criteria for success and failure differ from those of the medical community. Chapter 3 states that the goal of ministry is to bring people into God's own wholeness. Keeping that goal in mind removes the urge to obsess on results and helps us look beyond the present. Here, then, are three questions that teams should ask in judging the success or failure of their ministry:

1. Has God become real to the supplicant?

This is *the* key criterion. Often God is already real to a supplicant, but this question needs to be asked in reference to a particular ministry session. Making God real to a supplicant is why our ministry belongs in the category of worship instead of medical care. If God becomes experientially real, the ministry is a success. If God doesn't become more experientially real, the ministry is a failure. In other words, healing comes from God and should lead to God.

When God becomes real to supplicants, they grow in their personal relationship with their creator and savior. What previously may have been an intellectual assent to dogma becomes an intimate, *felt* encounter. Healing ministry that helps bridge the chasm between head and heart is always a success, even if nothing else appears to happen.

When supplicants have a personal encounter with God, they experience being cared for by him. They come to see themselves as beloved children of a benevolent creator. Regardless of any other tangible results, they lose their sense of isolation as they experience the reality of Jesus' promise: "I am with you always" (Mt 28:20b).

Often the experience of being cared for by God is mediated by the team. For instance, a woman named Ann had lost her voice in the aftermath of surgery on her vocal cords. After years of working in a dynamic nursing job that required much verbal communication, she felt despair at only being able to speak in whispers. The team treated Ann lovingly. First they listened to her frustration without dismissing it with cliches. (e.g., "You shouldn't feel that way." "These things take time.") They affirmed her for being a caring nurse even in the midst of her own medical problems. Then they prayed for God to cure her vocal cords. At the end of ministry, Ann asked, "Is this what God is like?" That's success.

Another sign of success in healing ministry is increased unity with the Body of Christ. Alienated Christians come back into their faith community, shut-ins feel less isolated, care-givers of shut-ins feel supported by their parish. Any time a prayer team draws these people into the Body of Christ, the ministry is a success.

2. Is the illness healed?

Chapter 3 covers the difference between healing illnesses and curing diseases. Healing ministry strives to heal illness, which is a person's *experience* of disease. Keeping this in mind, ministry succeeds if it increases a supplicant's hope and reduces his feelings of alienation that are the result of being sick. It also succeeds if it helps him sort out his feelings about having a disease.

Healing an illness may or may not include curing a disease. For example, ministry to Anthony did not result in his being cured of cancer. He died. But he was healed of the *illness* of having a terminal disease. Rather than viewing himself as just a dying person and a cancer patient, he grew to see himself as a devoted husband, father and grandfather as well as a vital member of the Body of Christ. And in the process of being ministered to for cancer, Anthony also experienced deep spiritual healing. He died closer to God than he had been prior to his illness.

3. Is the disease cured?

As described in Chapter 3, disease involves bodily organs. Overcoming disease can occur through physical, chemical, surgical, or, sometimes, prayer intervention. Healing ministry that locks itself into a focus on bodily organs loses sight of the whole person and of God. Success is seen as curing disease; failure is viewed as not curing disease. This leads to trying to *make* a cure happen. If Jesus had suffered from such spiritual near-sightedness, he would have set up health clinics throughout Israel instead of preaching the coming of the kingdom of God.

Diseases *are* cured through healing ministry; frequently this is an outcome of healing an illness. For instance, when Ann left the prayer team after her first session, her voice remained unchanged. During the next couple of months, however, she let go of her fixation on physical recovery. During a church service she silently asked God to be in control of her life, including her voice. As she began to relax, her vocal cords relaxed as well. Each time the prayer team saw her, she expressed more trust in God, more feelings of support by others and more willingness to release her demand for full recovery. By the end of two months of ministry, her voice had been restored. Her disease had been cured, primarily because her illness had been healed.

Sometimes a disease is not completely cured, but its symptoms abate, e.g., a supplicant with multiple sclerosis may go into remission for several years. Other times, a person being treated for, say, cancer, is freed from side effects of treatment such as chemotherapy. Still other times, a disease isn't cured but the supplicant experiences relief from pain. This can be especially liberating in the case of someone who is dying. Release from pain means release from mind-blurring drugs. Instead of vacillating between unspeakable pain and semi-consciousness, a dying person can spend his last days wrapping up his affairs and saying good-bye to loved ones.

Symptom abatement, freedom from side effects of treatment, release from pain: none of these is a "cure," but each is a form of healing. Each is a success.

Conclusion

Jesus failed in some of his healing ministry and so will we. In his healings he tried to lead people into an experience of God. Sometimes they missed it. For example, in the story of the ten lepers (Lk 17:11–19), ten people were cured, but only one was healed. Jesus' ministry to nine out of ten of the lepers was a failure because God hadn't become real to them. They only saw a change in their skin condition.

Ministry can be a success even in the absence of a cure. If we keep our eyes fixed on worship, we let go of "making" cures happen. Our focus changes from results to enabling people to grow into God's wholeness. Whenever we bring people into an experience of God's presence, our ministry succeeds, regardless of other outcomes.

Summary

Healing ministry is worship, and our goal as ministers is to create a worship experience for supplicants — to bring them into an awareness of God's presence in their need. Successful worship in healing ministry involves six ingredients:

1. Create a sacred space.

2. Gather as the Body of Christ.

3. Create an awareness of God's presence.

4. Focus on the supplicant's need.

5. Enter into the heart of worship.

6. Bring worship to a close.

When healing ministry is worship, our criteria for success and failure differ from those of the medical community. To evaluate ministry's success, we ask three questions (in descending order of importance):

1. Has God become more real to the supplicant?

2. Is the illness healed?

3. Is the disease cured?

Chapter Seven

Eight Pitfalls

What are the pitfalls that afflict ministers?

On a scale of one to ten, Jan's anxiety level scored an eight. She had received a phone call asking her to coordinate a satellite group for the Institute for Christian Ministries (ICM), and the call to leadership filled her with fear. Would she be a channel of God's grace, or would she "blow it"? How many damaging mistakes would she make? How tragic it would be to start out serving God, but end up harming the mission of Christ!

Jan's inner turmoil churned on until she sensed God making her a solemn promise: If she said yes to ministry, God *guaranteed* she would make mistakes, she would "blow it," she even, alas, would sometimes sin in this ministry. She also sensed, however, that God was bigger than her errors. Jesus could be Lord even of her mistakes.

The guarantee of errors didn't delight Jan. Nevertheless it relieved her of most of the performance pressure she then was feeling. The whole prayer experience deepened her trust in God. It gave her the grace to face ministry and say, "Your will be done, Lord."

Anyone who serves God can count on the humbling reality that people do make mistakes in ministry. Despite their best intentions, they do sometimes sin. Applying this unavoidable fact to our subject, this chapter describes eight pitfalls of the ministry of religious healing. Because no one has arrived at a state of divine perfection, *everyone* struggles with flaws in their ministry.

Our goal here is to warn you of the most common errors many have encountered in healing ministry so that you can exercise good discernment and bypass pits you never knew existed. We also present some thoughts on spiritual attitudes and practices that can help you deal with these problems. None of what follows is a formula ("Avoid this and you'll be a success!"). Instead, we offer observations from multiple prayer ministers who have been engaged in healing ministry since 1970.

1. Excessive Individualism

Lila (in Chapter 2) gradually slipped into a state of total individualism and isolation in ministry. She was a good person who became so immersed in herself and "her" ministry that she made disastrous errors that harmed some supplicants, including Henrietta.

Major symptoms: The major symptom of excessive individualism is a pulling away from church, from team ministry, from other ministers and, ultimately, even from God. Those who have stumbled into the pit of excessive individualism shun feedback from their faith community. They rely solely on a personal "hotline" to God that needs no input from others. Fully confident of the infallibility of that hotline, they invoke God's authority often in ministry, using expressions such as, "God told me . . ." and "God says here in the Bible . . . . " This leaves people fumbling for words — after all, who dares to disagree with God or with his word?

Excessive individualists subscribe to the Jesus-and-me spirituality we discuss in Chapter 2. Unfortunately, this approach carries the danger of eliminating even Jesus himself. Seen from the perspective of others, some may begin to act as if they were God. It's as though, having bestowed the gift of healing on someone, God excuses himself and goes on to other important matters. This person now has the gift of healing and can take over from there. Few are aware of God's absence in this pit because super-individualists sprinkle their conversations with the Lord's name.

The spirituality needed to avoid this pitfall: Chapter 2 gives a detailed description of a spirituality that can avert excessive individualism: a Christ/we, incarnational view that recognizes the presence of the risen Lord in the Body of Christ. Ministers of religious healing who develop a Christ/we spirituality value the discernment of other ministers, including that of church leaders. They often engage in team ministry within an ongoing faith community. Their ministry — and God's healing — flows from the Body of Christ.

2. Escapism

Erin knew prayer ministry from the giving side; she rarely experienced it from the receiving side. Now, however, she was teetering on the brink of burnout. While her husband spent every free moment basking in the glow of TV's light, Erin ran around doing household chores and parenting two teenage boys. The affirmation she received from the family seesawed somewhere between zero and miniscule. The only time they knew she existed was when she failed to provide some creature comfort they expected — dinner, clean clothes, transportation, whatever.

Erin slowly gave up expecting her family to meet any of her needs. If it hadn't been for her relationship with God, she would have escaped her loneliness by having an affair. Instead, she sought refuge in ministry. Here people valued her as an individual. Here she experienced the satisfaction of seeing people grow. Here she found an alternative family to the primary one that ignored her.

The happier that Erin became about her newfound affirmation, the grumpier Tom became. "Are you going out again?" he would growl, as she crossed his TV path on her way out the door. "You're never around any more." The kids echoed his complaints and started skipping school. Rather than confront these growing family problems, Erin escaped them by spending even more hours in ministry. To her dismay, however, the ministry didn't seem to benefit from her increased devotion. She began to feel burned out, both at home and in ministry. Finally, Erin sought help from a prayer team. "What's wrong?" she cried. "I'm serving God, yet my life is falling apart!"

People who are working the hardest at personal growth and caring ministry are the most likely candidates for escapism. The committed and the energetic fall into this pit, not the weak and the lazy. It's one of the most subtle, yet pervasive temptations that a minister of religious healing faces. Priests and religious succumb to escapism just as often as lay people.

Major symptoms: Escapists display a zeal for ministry in the midst of disintegrating or absent close relationships. Beneath these symptoms usually lurks a problem with individualism. Merits of personal achievement gradually turn into sins of self-interest. Is your spouse holding you back from ministry? Get divorced. Is your parish lifeless? Find another. Is your religious community cold and sterile? Leave it.

Our culture looks on individualism as a virtue. Frank Sinatra's "I Did It My Way" echoes through America, with scant help being offered for how to do it *our* way — in families, parishes and religious communities. Staring into society's void of support for long-term commitment and sacrifice, is it any wonder that devout ministers don't know how to nurture and value their close relationships? Many do not hear God's call to teeth-gritting faithfulness when every brain cell screams, "I quit!"

The spirituality needed to avoid this pitfall: The antidote to escapism is a passionate desire to do God's will. Judeo-Christian history overflows with stories of saints and prophets who developed this spirituality. Traditional Catholicism points to Mary and Joseph as role models for our journey into this no-holds-barred "yes."

Jesus, of course, is the ultimate example of someone with a passionate desire to do God's will. His words in the Garden of Gethsemane ("Let your will be done, not mine" [Lk 22:42]) show him doing God's will in the face of death. We may fantasize about doing likewise in dramatic settings, while day-to-day sacrifices leave us feeling peevish. Demanding children and unappreciative co-workers can cause us to forget that throughout his life Jesus maintained a passionate desire to do God's will in the midst of equally demanding and unappreciative people. He *lived* on God's approval: "My food is to do the will of the one who sent me . . ." (Jn 4:34a). We resist saying yes to God's will unless we come to know that God always seeks the very best for everyone, *including* us.

Those who commit themselves to developing a passionate desire to do the will of God should expect resistance. Our heritage as a nation has been to leave that which we do not like. On the surface, Americans look like conformists. They dress in the latest fashion, follow fads, and echo media messages. But the current of an individualistic "I gotta be me" spirit runs deeper, colder and stronger than cultural conformity. Today's role models sometimes stay and work things out when the going gets tough. Far more often, however, modern role models are escapists who leave loved ones while making such statements as, "I've got to find myself," or "I've got to serve the Lord, and you're holding me back, dear."

To offset society's messages of individualism, we need the Holy Spirit's gift of fortitude. Once we've discerned the Lord's will for us in a given situation, the gift of fortitude will give us the grace to endure in the presence of pain.

Knowing God's will through the process of discernment is no easy task! Church-sponsored training programs offer students the support of staff and peers in discerning to what level of ministry God is calling them. Small faith communities in parishes can provide similar help. The assistance of others is crucial for good discernment, since we can easily deceive ourselves through the strength of our feelings. Alone, we can plug our spiritual ears to the possibility that God's will for us in a painful spot *may* be to bring salvation to that situation. Yes, God may be calling us to leave, but on the other hand, he may be calling us to stay.

Erin's strong feelings had kept her from seeing her family clearly. After several months of ministry, she realized that God's will was for her to decrease her parish ministry and increase her home ministry. This meant confronting Tom with their need for marriage counseling. It meant getting the family to face their exploitation of her as a person. It also meant hounding the school and her teens until a good academic path had been rebuilt. But in the end, Erin matured into a more effective minister because her caring flowed out of the Body of Christ, a body that includes the family.

3. Lack of Prayer

Don's day got off to a poor start and went downhill from there. A warm bed lured him into hitting his alarm's snooze button three times too often. Exit morning prayer time and, consequently, his center of peace. Snarled traffic made him late for work, so he had to stay overtime to finish a project. This meant he was late for dinner and even later for his commitment to his parish's prayer ministry.

Don dashed in the door five minutes before the supplicant's scheduled arrival, and sank into the nearest chair. "What a day," he sighed. "Who is our supplicant? I can't remember who we saw last week." Don's team members looked at him in dismay. They had already been praying together for 25 minutes, asking the Lord to give them unity and all the spiritual gifts they needed for the evening's ministry. Now they were just finishing reviewing their previous week's ministry.

The results of Don's tardiness spilled over into ministry. Mentally he was still on the highway, so he couldn't bond with his team members. Having been absent during preparation for ministry, he had no idea what the team's discernment was for the supplicant.

Therefore, his contributions to the session bore no connection to everything else that was happening. At the end of the evening, the supplicant politely thanked the team for their prayers, but it was obvious to everyone that she had not had an experience of God during that hour. Like water escaping a leaky pipe, God's power was not reaching its intended source.

After several recurrences of the same scene Don told the team he didn't think God was calling him into ministry. He said his frazzled life led him to conclude that he was too busy to work both for the Lord *and* for a living. Furthermore, he didn't think he had the necessary gifts for being an effective minister. Why else would he have so little time and so few results? As he expressed these doubts to his teammates, one of them suggested he pray more about this before making any decisions about God's call to him. A sheepish look crossed Don's face. "Prayer?" he said. "Outside of ministry, I haven't done that for a while."

Major symptoms: The major symptoms of a lack of prayer are an absence of inner peace, a disunity with teammates, an inability to bring supplicants into God's presence, and ultimately, a lack of results in ministry.

Lack of prayer on the part of one team member impacts the entire prayer ministry. Unless it's dealt with, one person's problem becomes everyone's problem. Nevertheless, most of us squirm at the thought of asking others about their personal prayer life. In a country that genuflects to the right to privacy, questions about another's intimate relationship with God often feel invasive. Unless a person broaches the subject himself, we shy away from pinning someone down about how much daily time he's spending in private prayer.

If we don't feel comfortable asking team members direct questions about their prayer life, we must rely on symptoms. Are any teammates chronically late, often frazzled, lacking in fruit during ministry and lacking in team unity? Is there a team member who never talks about anything related to personal prayer? If one or more of these symptoms exists, this person may not be praying on a daily basis.

While lack of prayer is one of the hardest pitfalls to detect in others, it is one of the easiest to detect in ourselves. We need only ask if we are making daily, personal prayer a top priority. We cannot bring others into the healing presence of the Lord unless we ourselves regularly come into his presence! For ministers of religious healing, personal prayer underpins our entire ministry. Without it, everything we do sits squarely on a foundation of shifting sand. Also, without personal prayer, we're unlikely to intercede for our supplicants between sessions.

The spirituality needed to avoid this pitfall: Personal prayer is impossible without making it a priority. An extra half-hour of sleep in the morning will entrap us every day unless time with God becomes a higher priority than time in bed. Self-discipline is also a critical factor in personal prayer. A frantic, workaholic schedule can consume our lives unless we use daily discipline to find God's center of peace within ourselves.[1]

Daily prayer gives God enough space to reveal the level of ministry that's right for us. It gives us the ability to discern the difference between short-term time crunches and long-term commitments. Prayer gives us the courage to decide what goes and what stays. It gifts us with the ability to say "yes" to God's will. Best of all, personal prayer empowers us to engage in quality ministry within the Body of Christ.

In the aftermath of Don's admission that his personal prayer time had sunk to zero, the entire team decided they needed to develop guidelines for themselves. For instance, they could have avoided this problem altogether if each of them had made an initial, upfront commitment to daily prayer. Don's problem would have been recognized sooner if each week's preparation for ministry had been preceded by a few minutes' conversation about what was happening in everyone's personal prayer life. These moments could have lent the emotional support that people need to stay on a path of an ever deeper relationship with God.

As for Don, an earlier bedtime left him rested enough so he could quit wearing out the snooze button on his alarm. Centered in peace through prayer, he began to discern that his busy schedule did not allow time for the two prayer ministry sessions he'd been doing each week. But it did allow for one. On the day he engaged in ministry, he'd leave work a bit early, enjoy a quiet dinner and arrive rested and ready for ministry thirty minutes before the supplicant's arrival. While he was driving to work, he sometimes would say a rosary for the intention of the supplicant's healing. During ministry the prayer team's unity became a source of healing, and it enabled everyone — teammates and supplicant alike — to experience the presence of God.

4. Moralizing

Debbie gingerly sat down in the chair the prayer team offered her. She grimaced as muscles spasms rippled across her low back. "I'd like you to pray for healing for my back," she gasped. "This pain is killing me."

One of the team members, Agnes, knew Debbie personally. She knew she had married outside the church and had not been back since then. The team spent several minutes praying for Debbie's back, then Agnes started praying for her marriage. "Oh Lord," she began. "Forgive Debbie for marrying a non-believer." The prayer for repentance continued for several minutes, at the end of which time Debbie looked more like a victim of abuse than a recipient of ministry. It became obvious that the team was not achieving the results they wanted. In an effort to make Debbie deal with her spirituality, they dug themselves into a deeper hole by telling her God couldn't heal her back until she repented and returned to practicing her faith.

Needless to say, this prayer session reaped no benefits for Debbie. She arrived with one problem, low back pain, and left with two, low back pain and emotional pain. The latter drove her further away from dealing with her ongoing spiritual difficulties. She was not led into an experience of God that could heal both her body and her soul.

Major symptoms: Ministers of religious healing who moralize use prayer as a means of preaching. They appear to be praying to God when, actually, they are lecturing the supplicant. ("Oh Lord, we know that in Second Corinthians you tell us not to yoke ourselves to unbelievers. We thank you for our sister Debbie here, and we ask you to forgive her for committing this sin.")

Preaching-style prayer amounts to nothing less than spiritual mugging! Supplicants who might ward off criticism in a day-to-day setting have little or no barriers during prayer. In prayer, the ability to discard the bad and keep the good is radically diminished. Souls lie exposed before us. We ministers must acquire a profound reverence for that reality and develop a style of ministry whose hallmark is love and gentleness.

The spirituality needed to avoid this pitfall: The antidote to moralizing is trust in God — trust in his agape love for our supplicants and trust in his ability to lead them where he wants them to go. "Let God be God" sums up the spirituality we need for avoiding the pitfall of moralizing.

This is hard to do! As we gaze at someone in trouble and listen to God's apparent silence, the temptation is to succumb to worry. We fret about *how* God is going to work out his plan for a supplicant. We especially fret about salvation (the "salvation by interaction" described in Chapter 5). Anxiety creeps up and whispers to us that *we* are totally responsible for this person's salvation and healing. If we buy that message, it's good-bye loving ministers; hello worry-warts.

To let God be God, we need a clear understanding of our role in a supplicant's life. Preparation for ministry opens us to receive discernment about her readiness, about our abilities to be God's conduit, and about God's will for this session. Preparation gives us a road map for how far to go with our supplicant and how to get there.

Letting God be God leads us into a reverence for the sacredness of each person's spiritual journey. God does not expect people to leap tall buildings in a single bound! Rather, he leads them step by step on a holy journey toward the fullness of life. He asks us to accompany others on that path, often for only a few steps of the way. Because each step is crucial, our role is crucial. Without us, the next step may not happen. Nevertheless, we are never with others for their whole trip. We are not the Messiah who says, "I am with you always; yes, to the end of time" (Mt 28:20b). Realizing this fact can help us avoid moralizing and, instead, move us into humble trust. We join a brother or sister in Christ during a few steps of their journey toward the wholeness of God.

If Debbie's prayer team could have turned back the clock on their ministry, they would have spent the majority of their time praying for her back pain. At this point in her journey, she recognized God's possible role in physical healing. If the prayer team had honored Debbie's prayer request and trusted in God's power to work within that context, she might have been drawn toward other experiences of God beyond that ministry. At the end of the prayer session, the ministers could have invited their supplicant to try out the church again. ("Please come! We'd love to see you!") Invitations like this bear far more fruit than moralizing. They free people to say yes to God's will at each special moment in their lives. And they free us from the false responsibility of being pseudo-messiahs.

5. Advice-Giving

Alice wore an invisible "help me" sign. She shifted in her chair and avoided looking at the team members. "I'd like prayer for discernment," she said, clearing her throat. Then she described how her job didn't pay well, her boss treated her badly, and lay-offs loomed on the horizon. She knew of another job that involved more travel but better work conditions. "I want to know if I should take it," she ended.

Phil interjected that this reminded him of *his* past difficulties. "I faced the same decision several years ago," he said. As ten minutes ticked by, he proceeded to recount the ins and outs of his decision-making process and why Alice should do the same thing he did. Then Leslie said, "Phil, I disagree." Whereupon she listed all the reasons Alice should pray for her boss' healing, rather than job-hop. Exit another ten minutes. An argument ensued, with Phil and Leslie at loggerheads and Alice responding with "Yes, but. . ." followed by her litany of reasons why none of their suggestions would work.

Twenty minutes before the end of their hour together, the team finally entered into prayer, but by then no one was in a prayerful mood. The shortage of time did not enable them to re-establish the connection with God they had felt during preparation for ministry. Alice left the session with no peace, no answers and no discernment.

Supplicants like Alice are common. They ask for advice and we give it. As soon as we read their "help me" sign, we put on a matching one that says "I'll rescue you." Some supplicants *don't* ask for advice but we still give it; we supply the answer before the question is asked.

The urge to give advice can be as strong as an urge to cough. Some people's entire ministry consists of giving advice. Perhaps this is because this pitfall makes the *minister* feel better. We care deeply for people and long to relieve their pain. Not knowing exactly what to do, we resort to giving advice. It may not help, but we console ourselves with the thought that at least we're doing something.

Major symptoms: The major symptom of advice-giving is a ministry that's short on prayer and long on talk. One need only look at a watch to suspect the problem. It's distressingly easy to spend more time conversing with a supplicant than bringing that person into an experience of God through prayer. Personal stories like Phil's take the place of prayer. Certain phrases sprinkle the ministry: "Why don't you . . . . If I were you . . . ." And the ever-popular, "You should . . . ."

Spirituality needed to avoid this pitfall: As with the solution to moralizing, the way out of giving advice lies along the path of trust in God. This becomes possible if we maintain a focus on prayer and resist the desire to chat for long periods of time. A prayer focus gives us discernment as to what God wants for this person at this sacred moment in her spiritual journey, rather than what *we* want for her. It enables us to distinguish the subtle difference between instruction and advice. Finally, a focus on prayer helps us use the power of witnessing at the right time and place.

Trust in God leads us to the peaceful valley of humility, where we know who we are and who we aren't. We *aren't* rescuers who must solve all the problems of our supplicants. We *are* brothers and sisters in the Lord, called by God to travel a few steps with those who turn to us in need. Humility gives us the grace to place them before the Lord. We can join people like Alice at the foot of God's throne, where hearts are healed and courage is given. Witnesses of a birth, we stand in awe before the infinitely creative power of God.

6. Over-Identification

Ethel's husband, Roy, was drinking himself into unconsciousness every night and was in total denial about his alcoholism. After having gone to Al-Anon meetings for a year, Ethel finally decided to set up an "intervention" session with Roy — a carefully planned gathering of loved ones who would confront her husband about his disease. Ethel wanted the team to pray with her about her fears concerning the intervention.

As Ethel told her story, one of the prayer ministers began to feel angry. "That's not right!" Jill thought to herself. "*My* husband's an alcoholic, and I'm being patient with him. That's what the Lord tells wives to do!" These thoughts swirled through Jill's mind, turning her eyes inward toward the pain in her own marriage. Ethel's voice seemed farther and farther away, as did the entire ministry session. When one of team members asked Jill for some feedback about something that had just been said, she blinked as though they had just awakened her.

Major symptoms: When we over-identify with supplicants, their story pushes an internal button about *our* story. Ministry ceases as we become absorbed in our own pain. This robs us of the ability to help others.

When Jill over-identified with Ethel, she mentally withdrew, leaving the team with one less minister. Sometimes a minister doesn't withdraw; instead she becomes the supplicant by displaying an outpouring of emotion. She may cry and tell the supplicant she knows "just how he feels," but she's weeping about her own wounds, not his. Her behavior splits the ministry session in half because now there are two supplicants instead of one. The team faces a predicament; this is not the moment to minister to the minister, yet she is the one who is overwhelmed.

Spirituality needed to avoid this pitfall: Over-identification is a complex psychological problem with no easy answers. Ministers need to be emotionally whole enough to deal with other people's pain. If a supplicant's pain resembles a minister's own unhealed wounds, it will overwhelm the minister. In these cases, over-identification closes the door on that specific ministry until the minister has pursued further healing for himself.

Some doors, however, must remain closed. For example, sexual abuse victims often reach the point where they can minister very effectively to other sexual abuse victims. Rarely, however, can they tolerate prison ministry to sexual offenders. Some scars are too deep, and we must accept this reality. We can avoid feelings of failure by realizing that our God of mercy does not call us to be all things to all people.

Jill did not have to permanently close the door on ministry to supplicants impacted by alcoholism. But her reaction to Ethel showed her she needed to re-examine her handling of her husband's drinking. Experiences like Jill's are nearly universal in healing ministry: a supplicant's story uncovers an unsolved issue within us. We can look on this as an opportunity for further growth and healing for ourselves. It is an invitation from God.

7. Over-Timidity

When ICM (at the beginning of this chapter) asked Jan to coordinate a satellite, she had an acute attack of over-timidity. Feelings of inadequacy and the fear of making a mistake in ministry tempted her to say no to training people for prayer ministry. Over-timidity almost led her to say "no" to God's call to serve.

This pitfall has lots of company in scripture. All the prophets suffered from it at the start of their call. Jeremiah's response to his call is the cry of anyone caught in the grasp of over-timidity: "Ah, ah, ah, Yahweh; you see, I do not know how to speak" (Jer 1:6).

Major symptoms: The major symptom of over-timidity is not being involved in ministry. The absence of ministry may be total or it may be partial, such as avoiding ministry to some types of needs. For instance, many people feel unqualified to pray for someone seeking physical healing for a terminal illness. In the face of a life-and-death request, panic rises as mental tapes begin to turn: "I don't have the faith to do this! What happens if I pray and nothing happens?" As the supplicant sits before the team, performance pressure replaces peace because the team loses sight of God. The greater the pressure becomes, the less the ministry becomes, until soon prayers disintegrate into nervous babbling and the team vows that in the future they will avoid all prayer for physical healing.

A subtle form of over-timidity can be found in those teams who refuse to devise a plan of action for a prayer session during their preparation for that ministry.[2] "We don't want to stifle the Spirit," they say. But what they're really saying is "We're afraid to be wrong about our discernment of God's will for this supplicant in this session." Lacking strong but flexible plans of action, many prayer teams wonder why their ministry seems so wishy-washy and ineffective.

Over-timidity is a thin veneer which covers perfectionism. Jesus exhorts us to "be made perfect as your heavenly Father is perfect" (Mt 5:48, *NAB*). Here, Jesus is calling us to a lifelong spiritual journey, but often this verse feels like a condemnation of mistakes, especially mistakes in ministry. When we quake at the thought of divine disapproval of our errors, we can find quick relief from those fears by avoiding ministry altogether. Or, we can dodge discernment and leadership by adopting an unfocused style of ministry, "letting the Spirit lead" with little or no participation on our part.

Over-timidity obsesses on success. Knowing that every effort at ministry carries the risk of failure, we can wiggle free of this risk by saying: "Oh Lord, I am not worthy." Misused this way, this statement imparts a false sense of humility while releasing us from the responsibility to serve God. Of course we're not worthy! Of course we're incapable of doing a perfect job of ministry! Once we've acknowledged these facts, we can move on to a spirituality that frees us from over-timidity.

Spirituality needed to avoid this pitfall: The first thing we must know in order to avoid over-timidity is that ministry is not an option, it's an obligation. In the words of theologian Simon Tugwell:

> Just as the Father sent Christ, even so he sends us; and so we cannot opt out of the "greater works than these" which he promised us that we should do (Jn 14:12). Healing the sick, and casting out demons, and even raising the dead, are part of the job given to the church (Mt 10:8).... It is not for us to decide that we are unworthy to do such things. What makes us think ourselves worthy to do the things that we *do* do anyway? When St. Catherine said to the Lord on one occasion, "I am not worthy," he replied, "No, but I am worthy."[3]

This sort of statement can give rise to feelings of panic. How can we cope with our feelings of unworthiness and incompetence when confronted with such a challenging call? To do so, we need the gift of courage. Our new motto must become that of St. Paul: "There is nothing I cannot do in the One who strengthens me" (Phil 4:13). This belief kept Paul focused on doing great deeds for the Lord, despite his flaws. A gift from God gave him an insatiable hunger to serve the Lord. Theologians call this the gift of *magnanimity*.

Magnanimity feels like being irresistibly drawn toward ministry. Our free will remains intact, yet the desire to serve God is like an itch that won't subside until we scratch it. We *want* to engage in ministry, and we're willing to make sacrifices in order to do so. Magnanimity helps us overcome the natural tendency to shy away from doing difficult works of God. Fear of failure shrinks as the longing to serve grows.

But magnanimity requires a balancing virtue, or else it can warp itself into ambition and pride. St. Thomas Aquinas said magnanimity needs the companion virtue of humility:

> There is in man something great which he possesses through the goodness of God, and something defective which comes to him through the weakness of nature. Accordingly, magnanimity makes a man deem himself worthy of great things because of the gifts he has from God. . . . On the other hand, humility makes a man think little of himself in consideration of his own deficiency.[4]

Together, then, magnanimity and humility provide the balance that can make us hard working servants of the Lord. Humility allows us to acknowledge our limitations as a minister without becoming paralyzed, while magnanimity draws us into developing our gifts to their fullest. Humility keeps us grounded in a radical dependency upon God, while magnanimity gives us the boldness to "go out to the whole world; [and] proclaim the gospel to all creation" (Mk 16:15). Humility enables us to place our trust in a savior who can be Lord of our incompetence as well as our competence, while magnanimity empowers us to avoid over-timidity, confident that in Christ, we have strength for everything.

8. Pursuing Our Own Agenda

Nancy's marriage was in a state of collapse. Her husband, Frank, was an alcoholic who had immersed himself in a series of extramarital affairs, some with women, others with men. When finally he announced he wanted a divorce, Nancy felt crushed. As a Christian, she believed in the sanctity of marriage, yet she was suffering in an unfaithful, abusive relationship.

After weeks of agony, Nancy decided she could not surrender her belief in God's unwavering will for all marriages. She joined a group whose sole agenda was the saving of their marriages. Each week about a dozen people gathered to intercede for the salvation of their alienated partners and the resurrection of their defunct marriages. Even if a former spouse was happily remarried and a parent of small children, the prayers persisted. Even if someone had sexually abused his children, everyone believed the marriage should be restored.

Nancy's belief in the group was so strong that she convinced Frank to delay filing for divorce. "I stalled for time," she said, "so the prayers would have time to work." Intercession focused on "claiming" scripture verses that supported their position. One favorite: "Have respect for your own life then, and do not break faith with the wife of your youth. For I hate divorce, says Yahweh, God of Israel" (Mal 2:15b–16a).

Nancy's contact with the group lasted for six years, during which time some members sank into deep depression. Others dropped out. As for Nancy, she started feeling oppressed with guilt because she had lost her desire for God to save a destructive relationship. When she prayed for what she no longer wanted, she felt she was being dishonest with God.

Nancy's resolve finally snapped when Frank contracted gonorrhea and gave it to her. She began to have nightmares. If she could get gonorrhea, couldn't she also get AIDS? She decided to file for divorce. When Nancy broke the news that she had filed for divorce, the group told her that her decision was "not from the Lord." Then they coldly turned from her, making it clear they no longer wanted to associate with her.

Major symptoms: Single-minded rigidity is a major symptom of pursuing our own agenda. If we lock ourselves into one plan, one thought process, or one scripture verse, we tune out humanity as well as the fullness of God's will. Hurting people become nameless objects we use to fulfill our personal agenda. They become drums we can beat, violins we can play. By assaulting people in this fashion, we violate the sacredness of their journey with God.

Black-and-white thinking is another symptom of this pitfall. A man is saved or he's not. All marriages are permanent or none of them are. Everyone should be healed of all physical illnesses or the Bible has lied. This all-or-nothing mindset eliminates the need to consult God in each situation. Why seek God when we already know his thoughts? We can charge forth with scripture verses and/or church teaching because God has revealed his will to us, once and for all, and we need no further input.

Our own agenda always looks great on paper but often falls flat in real life. Jesus is a gentle, patient savior, but this pitfall removes sensitivity and timing, replacing it with the impatient *now* and the almighty *me*. For instance, if someone requests healing prayer for cancer, there's no doubt that now is the time for this healing to occur, and I am the one to make it happen. This style of ministry often fails to bear fruit. That should be our clue that we may be pursuing our own agenda.

It has been our observation that group dynamics can play a part in this pitfall. In Nancy's case, the whole group propped each other up with their conviction that the Lord would restore each of their failed marriages. Alone, few of the members would have had the strength to endure. Together, how could they all be wrong? On prayer teams, if one person has a personal agenda, usually he has the strength to cling to it because of the invisible support of a group he has encountered elsewhere. The support group may be nothing more than a TV evangelist with a dynamic, unbending message, but the prayer minister grips onto this as proof of the correctness of his convictions.

A team member with a personal agenda can wreak havoc on a prayer team and on a supplicant, especially if he pursues his goal in a forceful or condemning manner. The team probably will break up because of the one member's rigidity. But if it permits him to continue this style of ministry, or even joins him in it, the supplicant will be badly damaged. It is a devastating experience for a supplicant when a team misuses the power of community by ganging up on her. If she lacks the strength to withdraw from ministry, the abuse will be magnified. Her spiritual journey will stop, not advance. It may take years for her to recover from the trauma of bad ministry.

Spirituality needed to avoid this pitfall: To avoid this problem, we need a passionate desire to learn. The relentless pursuit of a personal agenda must be replaced by a no-holds-barred openness to God, to supplicants, to the Body of Christ and to life in general. In short, we must be teachable.

When we are teachable, we open ourselves to endless options for ministry. This openness stands on a foundation of reverence for the *fullness* of God's will in every human life. As described in Chapter 3, God's plan for supplicants is their ultimate sharing in his wholeness. Our striving for one isolated agenda item pales when placed next to this goal.

Openness leads us to respect the sacredness of people's free will. God's finest plans for Nancy's marriage may have been for Frank to seek treatment for alcoholism, repent of adultery, and be healed of his need for promiscuity. But God never violates our free will, even to achieve a positive goal. To do so would destroy our identity as children of God and turn us into slaves.

When we are teachable, we acquire the art of timing. Many a ministry opportunity has been ruined by vaulting over God's specific desire for a supplicant and trying to force him to instantly accept God's long-range plan. We may know a man's problem arises from, say, selfishness, but until the time is right for him to see this fact, he won't be able to be healed. Cramming repentance down his throat at the wrong time will only alienate him from the Body of Christ and from God. It will slow his healing, not assist it.

Finally, when we are teachable, we grow in wisdom and knowledge through study as well as through experience. People who believe they've "arrived" in any situation, be it in ministry, relationships, or life, ultimately become pathetic shells of what God would like them to be. By turning their acquired knowledge into a god, they slam the door on the additional knowledge that lies before them. They become living examples of an old expression: "Start me right, I never change."

For our ministry to blossom, then, we must set aside our own agenda and constantly open ourselves to learning. It took six years for Nancy to realize that neither she nor Frank had had the maturity or wholeness to marry each other in the first place. Prior to their marriage, they both had needed healing. While Nancy had grown and sought healing during her marriage, Frank had acted out his woundedness through drinking and promiscuity. Her increased wholeness clashed with his continued pain, until both were caught in a whirlpool of destruction. After their divorce, Nancy met a devout Christian, an elder in her church. Today, Frank maintains his self-destructive lifestyle, but Nancy now is happily remarried and sharing in ministry with her new husband.

Conclusion

Today's ministers must be psychologically whole in order to resist the power temptations that come with healing ministry. Many people are attracted to this field because they are *not* emotionally well; without meaning harm, they create more pain than they alleviate. Most pitfalls in ministry relate at least partially to psychological health.

> Psychological health in ministers is not a luxury. Some optional ways of living — deeply neurotic, addictive — are not suitable. . . . False ministry reveals itself as an immature or neurotic will to replace the divine or to engage in a self-serving charade. . . . Of all human endeavors religion is particularly susceptible to neurosis. . . . [5]

Having said that, we must add that ministers who place themselves at God's service *do* fall temporarily into most of these pits. Leo recently asked an experienced prayer minister how many of these eight ministry mistakes she and her prayer partner had ever made. "We've made 'em all," she said. If you find yourself giving the same answer to the same question, then welcome to the Body of Christ, a community of believers whose God is mightier than anyone's errors.

The usual scenario for dedicated ministers is: They make a mistake; they realize their error; they feel humiliated at seeing their imperfections and limitations; and finally, they emotionally beat themselves up for having "blown it." But this is *not* God's reaction to our mistakes. When we make errors in ministry, God does not condemn us, nor does he want us to condemn ourselves! Instead, the Lord calls us to come to terms with our failures without being overwhelmed by them. He wants us to look on these experiences as opportunities for learning and growth, paths for moving into deeper, better and more humble ministry.

When we persevere in the ministry in spite of failure, we eventually grasp the amazing truth of Romans 8:28 — God turns the bad of our errors into good. We learn from mistakes and become stronger because our ministry is grounded in the kind of wisdom only experience can give. We grow in the humility that comes from totally depending on God's power working through us.

> (God) has answered me, "My grace is enough for you: for power is at full stretch in weakness." It is, then, about my weaknesses that I am happiest of all to boast, so that the power of Christ may rest upon me; and that is why I am glad of weaknesses.... For it is when I am weak that I am strong (2 Cor 12:9–10).

By seeing our startling capacity to blunder, we acquire the compassion that arises from having walked in the shoes of failure. This gives us a sure-fire antidote to being judgmental and condescending with supplicants. Wearing the shoes of failure for a while gives us the gift of empathy, a fundamental trait needed for the ministry of religious healing.

Wisdom, humility, compassion, empathy. We find these virtues in the school of ministerial experience. In this school, one fact consoles us when we blunder: God always shows up! He never fails to be present in ministry. That's why we have the courage to say, "I have come to do your will, O God" (Heb 10:7, *NIV*).

Summary

Pitfalls	Major Symptoms	Spirituality Needed
1. Excessive individualism	Isolation, rejection of input from others, Jesus-and-me spirituality	Christ/we spirituality (see Chapter #2 summary for details)
2. Escapism	Zeal for ministy with disintegrating or absent close relationships	A passionate desire to do God's will, assistance of others to discern God's will
3. Lack of Prayer	Absence of inner peace, disunity with teammates, inability to bring supplicants into God's presence, lack of results in ministry	Discipline in one's spiritual life, making prayer a top priority
4. Moralizing	Being judgmental or preachy, especially using prayer to preach	Trust in God, "letting God be God," reverence for the sacredness of each person's spiritual journey
5. Advice-giving	Ministry that is short on prayer, long on talk; attempting to solve others' problems for them	Trust in God, developing humility to recognize Jesus as Lord
6. Over-identification	Total absorption in supplicant's immediate pain; cessation and/or avoidance of some types of ministry; reversal of roles, minister suddenly becoming the supplicant	The virtue of hope, ability to focus outward and to keep God's "big picture" in mind, getting one's own woundedness healed

Pitfalls	Major Symptoms	Spirituality Needed
7. Over-timidity	Non-ministry, perfection-sim, refusal to devise a plan of action for ministry sessions, obsession with need to succeed	Magnanimity (insatiable hunger to serve God) plus humility
8. Pursuing one's own agenda	Single-minded rigidity, black-and-white thinking, poor timing, lack of fruit in ministry	Desire to learn, teachability, reverence for the fullness of God's will in every life, respect for the sacredness of supplicant's free will

Chapter Eight

The Spirituality of the Supplicant

How does the spirituality of a hurting person (supplicant) impact healing ministry?

One premise of this book is that life is a spiritual journey. Everything we do, say or think contributes to or detracts from progress on this journey. If religious healing is a transformation into God's wholeness (Chapter 3), then seeking that healing is a religious act. This chapter describes the search for God and his wholeness through the process of religious healing.

Dorothy's Story

To protect confidentiality and allow us to freely describe the inner dynamics of a supplicant's spiritual journey, we've created a composite account of ministry. Dorothy Knight does not literally exist, although prayer ministers encounter many Dorothys. Her healing illustrates the issues, feelings, struggles and victories that ministers of religious healing regularly encounter. We use journal entries to convey thoughts.[1] Throughout the chapter, we periodically comment on key points regarding the spirituality of the supplicant.

April 10:   Black, black, black, black, black — it's no use. Even if I wrote it a hundred times, it still wouldn't say how black it is down here. I'm at the bottom of a pit. It feels like I've been down here forever. I can't get out because this pit is so deep and there's no ladder or anything. I can look up and see light. Everybody's up there in the light, and I'm trapped

115

down here alone. Sometimes I feel like screaming "Help me! Help me!" But then I don't because it's no use — nobody can understand. Besides, nobody can help me because nobody can change the past.

Every morning I wake up and say, "God, how can I get out of here? I'm so worn out. I don't know where to turn. What can I *do*?" But God doesn't answer. He's *very* displeased with me. Ha! Forget that "displeased" junk. He's condemned me. I know that because he's been punishing me now for over a year. What I wonder is, why did God make me in the first place, when he knew I was going to end up in hell? In grade school the nuns used to say, "We're sinners, but God loves us anyway." But some sins are unforgivable. Once you've committed one of those, you can forget about the rest of your life. You might as well die and go to hell and get it over with.

I feel like I'm being sucked into death — it's my only way out. This pain is worse than childbirth. There's no relief! Somebody help me! But everyone is up there in the light, and I'm down here in the dark. Nobody can reach down this far. I'm scared because I'm going to die.

April 30:   I've been sitting here for hours trying to decide how I'm useful to anyone, and I can't think of *one* thing. Actually, I've been useless all my life. The world would be better off without me because I'm a burden to everyone. Really, I'd be doing everyone a favor if I killed myself.

Maybe my family will feel bad for a while, but Frank deserves a better wife. And Tom and Jennifer are almost out of their teens. They say things like "Mom, you don't know anything," or "I can't stand the way you dress these days. You embarrass me." Secretly, they'll be *relieved* to have me out of their hair!

And Caitlin — she's so young that after a month or two, she won't remember me. She's been crying in her crib for over an hour now, but I can't bring myself to go in and pick her up. Frank will remarry after I die. His new wife will love Caitlin more than I can.

How can I do this without making a disgusting mess? It has to be tidy. But mostly, it has to *work*. If it doesn't work the first time, it'll create a big commotion. Then I'll be *more* of a burden than ever.

Probably pills will be simplest. Some night when Frank is working late, I'll swallow a bunch of sleeping pills and go to bed early. He won't notice I'm dead until he comes to bed after the eleven o'clock news.

Ever since Caitlin's birth, Frank had been worried about Dorothy's behavior and had tried to talk with her about his concerns, but each time she simply had said, "It's no use talking about it. I'm sorry I'm not a good wife and mother." Finally, in mid-May Frank sat down and said, "Look, dear, I *know* something is wrong. You used to dress well. Now you stay in your bathrobe all day. You used to love cooking, and now you can't even stand to buy food. I love you, and I'm really worried about you. You seem so terribly unhappy these days."

Frank refused to end the conversation when Dorothy gave her standard answer to his concerns. After fifteen minutes, she started crying and told him she felt so low she wanted to die. When he realized she was having suicide thoughts, he said they needed to find a good psychiatrist for her. This made her weep all the more. "You think I'm crazy. I'm *not* crazy — I just can't stand this pain anymore. And besides, psychiatrists cost a ton of money."

> *June 1:* My birthday. People have been wishing me a happy birthday, but I don't think I'll ever feel happy again. Frank found a psychiatrist that he says can help me. Ha! If Dr. Robinson *really* knew me and the terrible thing I did, he'd know that I *am* hopeless. But I'm not going to tell him about it, just like I've never told Frank or anyone else. But *God* knows and now he's punishing me for what I did. He made me get pregnant with Caitlin. Then he gave her a huge birthmark that covers half of her face. Why do such a cruel thing to an innocent child? *She* isn't the one who sinned — *I* am. Every time I look at Caitlin's face, I see my soul — ugly and red.
>
> Yesterday I saw Dr. Robinson for the first time. I expected him to make me lie down on a couch and "free associate," just like they talked about in my Psych 101 class. Instead, he asked me to tell him what's happening these days. I told him about Caitlin and her birthmark. I said I feel bad about it, but I didn't tell him that *I'm* to blame.
>
> Dr. Robinson asked if I'd be willing to take antidepressants. I went along with him. I didn't have the nerve to ask if he

was prescribing an "upper." I never tried those when I smoked marijuana in college. Who knows? Maybe pills will give me enough energy to do *something* around here. This place is a mess.

The Knights' flower beds had taken on the appearance of a vacant lot. Usually Dorothy made them a showplace. She and a neighbor, Judy, normally chatted together while they tackled weeds in their yards, but now Dorothy stayed inside with her drapes drawn. One day Judy stopped by with a sack of plums from her backyard tree. Dorothy came out and sat with her on the front steps, saying she couldn't invite anyone inside because the house was a mess. When Judy said she missed their garden chats, Dorothy confided that recently she'd been feeling too low to do anything. During the next couple of months, she gradually opened up during Judy's brief visits, until finally she revealed that she was seeing a psychiatrist. "He's given me some medicine. I think it's making me feel a bit better."

Judy knew that Dorothy was Catholic. Eventually she broached the subject of a Catholic prayer team that ministered to people that needed healing. "I think you'd find it helpful. The people would pray with you for whatever you'd like."

August 15:   Judy has come up with the craziest idea I've ever heard — she thinks a *prayer* team might make me feel better! She's not Catholic, so she doesn't know I can't go to communion any more. Tom and Jennifer say it's "weird" to have a mother who goes to mass every Sunday but doesn't go to communion. I just tell them that's my business, not theirs.

A zillion questions pop into my mind when I think about this prayer team idea, and I fired off most of them at Judy. Do these people get carried away? If I did do this, would I be trapped? I wonder what they (and Judy) would think if they *really* knew.

Judy's neat — she's a better friend than I deserve. She answered all my questions. Then she gave me the phone number of one of the team members. She said this woman, Suzanne, can tell me more. Why should I call? If God is punishing me, how could they help? On the other hand, maybe they're like Judy. She makes me feel less alone, and she never gives me advice — thank God for that!

August 22: I had the strangest experience this morning: I was standing in front of our living room window looking at the sunrise and thinking about my situation. Suddenly a thought popped into my head: "It's time to grow up." How bizarre — where did that thought come from? I'm 40 years old and I'm not grown up? What have I been doing all these years? And what does it mean to "grow up"? I wonder if a prayer team could give me a few clues. *Maybe* I'll call them.

A few days later, Dorothy steeled her nerves, phoned Suzanne and learned that if she didn't like what went on, she could leave at any time. Suzanne said that most people try ministry for one session and then decide if they want to return. She also explained some of the process of ministry. At the end of the conversation, Dorothy said, "I guess I'll come just once and see what I think." She scheduled an appointment.

Comment: Healing is a journey that begins long before a prayer team ever meets a supplicant. Every journey is initiated by God, who uses a variety of means to invite someone to new life, to *conversion*. He provides the grace that is needed to respond to his invitation. In the words of St. Paul, "It is God who, for his own generous purpose, gives you the intention and the powers to act" (Phil 2:13).

Conversion goes beyond a single event. It is like marriage — a lifetime of incidents consisting of a few peak experiences and a multitude of daily little "yeses." The relationship a couple needs for a strong marriage starts in their courtship, increases with their engagement, and moves into the peak experience of their wedding day. Then begin years of fidelity, work, joy, suffering, and sharing, thousands of yeses in a shared journey through life. The wedding day is essential because without it no marriage exists. But the wedding day isn't the whole marriage.

Conversion begins with a person's recognition that he needs to change in some way — behavior, attitudes, health, religious denomination, relationships, etc. Many events build up to the moment when a vague awareness becomes a conscious thought. Something clicks. In Dorothy's case, a late pregnancy triggered depression and guilt about a past sin. Intervention by her husband, a psychiatrist, a neighbor, and even nature (the sunrise) brought her to the moment when she suddenly realized she needed to "grow up." God's invitation to conversion and his grace to say yes were mediated through people, nature, and circumstances.

Conversion and healing are as intertwined as threads in a tapestry. Those who refuse the former cannot experience the fullness of the latter. This is one reason that healing often fails to occur, both in medical and religious circles. Millions of people need healing from some problem or illness, but only a fraction of them are *motivated* enough to take the journey towards wholeness.

Some people deny the existence of their problem, as with a smoker who says his cigar-chomping grandfather lived to be 90. Conversion would lead him to "choose life" (Dt 30:19) in terms of his long-term health. Other people resist conversion by denying their need for help from anyone. For instance, a woman may assert that when she accepted Jesus as her savior, he completely healed her of cancer. Even continued symptoms may not budge her belief that she needs no more treatment, no prayer ministry, no more medication.

Some people avoid conversion because of feelings of low self-worth. Dorothy felt she deserved her suffering; God was punishing her. This belief initially blocked her from phoning the prayer team. And some people avoid conversion because they like the role of being ill. Secondary gains such as extra attention make it more pleasant for them to be ill than to be well.

Finally, a number of people simply aren't willing to put out the energy it takes to journey towards wholeness. Conversion and religious healing are hard work! God asks a lot from those who seek healing. He wants their hearts, their time, their courage, their energy, and their very lives. The magnitude of this task is why the Body of Christ plays such a crucial in its success. Just when a supplicant's energy and courage are at their lowest, others must help strengthen what is weak.

Dorothy's healing would have been blocked if she had refused to receive the help that was offered to her. She could have stuck with her standard answer to Frank when he again brought up the subject of her changed behavior. She could have balked at taking the prescribed antidepressants. She could have slammed the door in Judy's face, or rejected the idea of prayer ministry. Instead, Dorothy *cooperated* in her own healing.

Cooperative supplicants have overcome one of the greatest obstacles to the spiritual journey: a fear of loss of autonomy, of independence. The anxiety can be summed up in one basic question: If I let others into my life, will I still be me? It is especially prominent in those who seek healing. Dorothy expressed it as "will I be trapped?" She risked giving up some control if she revealed herself to others. This demanded a high degree of *trust*, both in God and in people. When looking at the magnitude of this risk, perhaps the wonder is not that so few people take the journey towards wholeness, but that so many do.

Prayer Ministry: Beginnings

To calm Dorothy's fears, Judy asked her if she'd like a ride to her first prayer ministry session. She accepted the offer. Suzanne greeted them on their arrival and invited them both into the ministry room, where everyone introduced themselves. Then Judy excused herself, telling Dorothy she would be waiting for her in another room.

This particular team had three members: Mary (the team leader), Suzanne, and Ruth. After explaining the basic process of ministry and reassuring Dorothy that they wanted to do only what she felt comfortable with, Mary asked her what she thought her most pressing need was, as of that moment. She said she felt very depressed. "Oh, that's a lonely place to be, isn't it?" responded Ruth. Dorothy nodded, fighting back tears. She and the team sat in silence for a minute, absorbed in that loneliness. When Mary asked when the depression began, Dorothy said it began when she got pregnant, but got much worse after the baby was born.

The team spent half of the first ministry session listening to Dorothy so as to discover what circumstances and issues were impacting her life. They found out that Caitlin was an unplanned, mid-life baby with a strawberry birthmark. Whenever Caitlin was out in public, strangers would shatter Dorothy with their comments, e.g., "Are there other people in your family who are marked like that?" "How come you don't do anything about that?" "Oh, the *poor thing*." In response to this insensitivity, Dorothy now was hiding the baby from society. Both she and Caitlin had become prisoners in their own home.

Prayer during this first session included affirming Dorothy for her openness in sharing about Caitlin and about her feelings. They thanked God for the gift of life he'd given to Dorothy and to Caitlin, and they asked him to begin to lift Dorothy out of her depression and to shower his love down upon her. Then the team sought feedback from her and asked her if she wanted to return. When she said "yes," they made an agreement with her to spend the next several sessions praying for healing from depression, especially as related to the baby.

Sept. 15: Yesterday I had my second session with the prayer team. These are *very* loving people. I wonder if they'd be shocked at anything I said. In the first session I said that when I got pregnant, I didn't want the baby. Then I said I felt like a babysitter, not a mother — I couldn't seem to feel any *love* for Caitlin. The team didn't faint. Instead, they understood, and still seemed to love me! That blew me away. No one in my life has ever loved me when I told them bad things. For sure, my folks never did. Maybe Frank would if I chanced it, but I can't. If he stopped loving me, that would be the end.

I almost had to back out of yesterday's session. Just before I was supposed to leave, Sally phoned to say she couldn't sit for Caitlin because she was sick. So I called Judy. She said why not bring the baby with us and she'd take her for a walk during my session. Secretly, I was afraid to have the team see Caitlin. But I couldn't see any way out, so that's what we did.

I cringed when Mary, Suzanne, and Ruth first laid their eyes on Caitlin. "Oh Lord, help me bear this," I thought. Then the team started oohing and ahhing over Caitlin, just like she was normal! They didn't seem to see the birthmark. Instead, they saw a baby. Then *I* began to see her too. How amazing! I've had a baby for nine months now, and all I've ever seen before was her birthmark! I started crying because for the first time ever, I felt some love for Caitlin. The team held her and they held me. Then they anointed both of us and prayed for God to bond us to each other. By the time they were done with that, everyone was crying! I feel like a weight has lifted from me. Last night I rocked Caitlin to sleep. It felt good.

Comment: Healing nearly always occurs within a climate of some heightened emotion — tears, joy, love, relief, etc. The emotions vary in intensity, depending on personalities and the type of healing involved. Like a fire that needs both oxygen and fuel for its existence, healing needs heightened emotions. Psychiatrist Jerome Frank states it this way:

> All forms of therapy, when successful, arouse the patient emotionally. The role of emotional arousal in facilitation or causing therapeutic change is unclear. One can only note that it seems to be a prerequisite to all attitudinal and behavioral change. It accompanies all confrontations and success experiences . . . . [2]

Part of Dr. Frank's research on the role of emotions in healing included studying cures at the shrine of Lourdes. There he discovered that " . . . Persons who remain entirely unmoved by the ceremonies (at Lourdes) do not experience cures."[3]

For healing to take place, then, supplicants need a *willingness to experience emotions*. A primary one that supplicants report is a sense of personal closeness with God and with ministers. In the second session, Dorothy experienced love, the feeling of a weight lifting from her, intimacy with Caitlin and closeness to the prayer team. Through the team, she also experienced God's love, but she was not yet aware of that fact.

Some supplicants are willing to experience emotions, including God's love, but just from God himself. They want help, but only via a direct hotline to the Lord. This Jesus-and-me spirituality (Chapter 2) denies the presence and healing power of Christ in his Body. Ministry in these cases cannot succeed because the prayer team is superfluous. Those who believe that the grace of Christ is unmediated do not need mediators, i.e., people. Fortunately, Dorothy did not have this problem. She was *open to receiving help from God through people* — through her psychiatrist, her family, her neighbor, and her prayer team.

To receive help from God through a prayer team, supplicants must have the *ability to establish a committed relationship with the team.* Dorothy's effort to resolve her last-minute schedule problem revealed that this was no casual, "if-I-have-nothing-better-to-do" commitment. She wanted to keep her appointment with the team and refused to withdraw at the first sign of difficulty. This is not a given in prayer ministry. Failure to show up for ministry will doom it from the start.

Part of any committed relationship is *self-disclosure*, the willingness to give another person knowledge about oneself. This is risky business because knowledge confers power, and sometimes that power is abused. When Dorothy revealed that she didn't feel love for Caitlin, the team could have misused this information by, for instance, disapproving of her or talking outside of ministry about her lack of love. Instead they treated her self-disclosure in the way that ministers must treat such knowledge: as a sacred treasure that belongs only to the supplicant and God.

Nothing will destroy healing ministry faster and more surely than violating the need for self-disclosure to be kept confidential! This holds especially true for parish-based ministry, where everybody knows everybody. If confidentiality is breached even *once* with *one* person, then a supplicant's self-disclosure becomes fuel for a gossip machine. Ministers of religious healing must make a specific verbal agreement with a supplicant that nothing said in the ministry will leave that room, and then they must *stick with that agreement*!

Self-disclosure is essential for a supplicant's spiritual journey because it helps him make sense of what has been, and is, happening to him. In naming and revealing his feelings and struggles, he gains some control over them. Alcoholics Anonymous makes good use of this. A key moment in a drinker's recovery takes place when he can stand up at an AA meeting and say, "My name is Joe, and I am an alcoholic." The disease is named. Now it can be dealt with as an objective reality.

> *Sept 22:* Yesterday I took a chance and showed the team last week's journal entry. They thought it was super. When we got into prayer, they thanked God for giving me the courage to share my journaling with them. They also thanked him for my having the gift of trust in them as a team. It's funny. I never knew that courage and trust were gifts from God. I thought they were attitudes I had to dredge up by myself.
>
> Is it possible that if I ask God for what I need, like courage and trust, he will give it to me? That sounds passive, and I'm discovering that getting out of this pit is anything but passive. For instance, Dr. Robinson says that antidepressants won't solve all my problems. I need therapy too. In my sessions, he keeps asking me how I *feel* about things. When I say "depressed," he says "look deeper." He's right about one thing: depression is like a blanket that smothers lots of other feelings. I need to lift up the corner of this mangy cover and peek under it. But I'm scared. What if the feelings that lie beneath it are even uglier than the blanket itself?

Prayer ministry isn't all that passive either. Mary tells me I'm a part of the team, a vital member. Life would be so much simpler if I could sit like a statue of the Blessed Mother while the team "prayed over me." I wouldn't need to *do* a thing. In a flash, God would do everything. Zap! and I'm well. Wouldn't that be nice?

Ruth says healing is a journey, and that's the way it's beginning to feel. It would be easy if I were going to Europe, but I'm not — I'm going inside myself. There's no way I could do this alone. This would be too scary without help. The prayer team and Dr. Robinson all seem like safe, strong people who are *with* me on this journey. But one question keeps gnawing at me: Would they stay with me if they knew the horrible thing I did in college? I *long* to get this off my chest, but what will they think of me if I tell them?

Comment: A supplicant must be an *active participant* in her healing, a process that includes every level of her being: physical, emotional, spiritual, and relational. Woundedness has made her dysfunctional in at least one of these areas, and healing the wounds will require great energy. Years of pain do not vanish like magic. Instead, pain peels away like layers of an onion, and the act of peeling entails work on everyone's part: supplicant, ministers, and God. Some supplicants say it resembles giving birth.

Participating in one's own healing means taking action wherever and whenever it's needed, e.g., praying during the week, reading, changing external circumstances, changing relationships, receiving the sacraments, taking part in the life of a faith community, etc. In Dorothy's case, journaling and therapy reinforced and strengthened what occurred during prayer ministry. Her efforts meant that healing could take place twenty-four hours a day, instead of one hour a week.

Prayer teams sometimes encounter a supplicant who expects the ministers to be "healers" who do all the work while he does all the receiving. Ministry in this situation rarely succeeds because it excludes the very person who needs healing. A passive supplicant is like a starving person who sits down at a lavish banquet and says to the other guests, "You eat, I'll watch."

Passivity in healing ministry allows the supplicant to see himself as helpless. He's been victimized by the past and is doomed to be victimized in the future. This was the attitude of the man whom Jesus cured at the Pool of Bethesda (Jn 5:1–15):

> . . . "Do you want to be well again?" "Sir," replied the sick man, "I have no one to put me into the pool when the water is disturbed. . . ." Jesus said, "Get up, pick up your sleeping-mat and walk around" (Jn 5:6–8).

Jesus had to rouse the man to *action* in order for healing to occur. Today's prayer ministers encounter this same challenge. (Chapters 9 and 10 explore this in greater depth.)

Some supplicants are willing to be active participants in their healing, but are adamant that they only need healing for one problem. This may be true, and ministers must respect an initial prayer request and focus their ministry on that need. But one wound often leads to another. A straight-forward problem may cloak a deeper one. At this point, supplicants face a choice: Do they just want to shed their current pain, or are they willing to embark on a spiritual journey and go wherever God leads them? Most people, such as Dorothy, start the healing process as a way to get out of pain ("Zap! and I'm well"). How far they advance beyond that target depends on their courage, the time and ministry that's available to them, and the grace of God.

The journey toward wholeness does deal with a supplicant's original problem. If it needs to go deeper than that, it will change his beliefs, his habitual ways of responding to stress, and his view of the meaning of his life. What starts as, say, knee pain, may lead a supplicant into the center of his being.

Prayer Ministry: Moving Into Deeper Issues

Each time the prayer team met with Dorothy, they sensed that she was moving into deeper trust in them and in God. She sat with a less guarded posture than at first. She responded to their questions more openly, without weighing each word ahead of time. And she shared many of her journal entries with them.

One day Dorothy came to ministry in an obvious state of agitation — guarded, on the verge of tears, pausing before saying each word. Seeing this, the team started the session by focusing on peace. After ten minutes, Dorothy said she had decided to show them a journal entry, and then read her September 22nd entry to them. When she got to the end and read "I *long* to get this off my chest, but what will they think of me if I tell them?" she began to sob. Suzanne put her arm around Dorothy and gave her some tissues. Ruth and Mary began to pray softly.

After a minute, Suzanne said, "It is really difficult to trust anyone this much." Dorothy nodded. The team spent the next several minutes responding with empathy to Dorothy's struggle. Finally she said she needed to tell them about college. She told them about leaving home as a "good girl" who had never made a ripple of trouble for anyone. Throughout her freshman year at the University of Iowa, she attended mass faithfully and was active in the Newman Club. But in her sophomore year she met a student named John who called himself a hippie. He introduced Dorothy to drugs, sexual activity, and "freedom from religion." Her parents were dismayed about their daughter's new lifestyle, but John said they were a couple of "fossils" who didn't know what life was all about.

In her junior year, Dorothy discovered she was pregnant. Suddenly she felt trapped in a vice, squeezed between her current lifestyle and her good-girl past. Her biggest fear was that her parents would "kill her" if they found out she was pregnant. John said they would never know about it if she got an abortion. He said abortions were "no big deal." An earlier girlfriend of his had had one. He would pay for it and no one would ever know. In a state of panic, Dorothy agreed to his plan and obtained an abortion.

Weeping profusely, Dorothy told the team her life had never been the same after that. She and John soon broke up because every time she saw him, it reminded her of what she'd done. She returned to church but never to the sacraments because she felt her sin was unforgivable. Her recent, unexpected pregnancy reawakened memories of the abortion. And when Caitlin was born with a large birthmark, she felt she was to blame.

> *October 15:* I did it. I told them. I couldn't stand to do it, but I did it anyway. Oh God, I feel so much *better.* Someone else knows, and they don't condemn me. They heard what I said and still love me. They didn't *excuse* what I did, but they understood the horrible bind my college pregnancy put me in.
>
> Mary says I can be forgiven. Is this *true*? Ruth and Suzanne agree with Mary. Suzanne has written down a scripture verse for me: "So confess your sins to one another, and pray for one

another to be cured" (Jas 5:16). I read it every time I think I can't be forgiven. It's a good thing they wrote this out for me — my old Bible is buried somewhere in the basement.

So the "healing" I need is forgiveness. That reminds me of the old days of going into the "black box" with a shopping list of sins. The team says that's not what they're talking about here. They say my telling them about the abortion was a type of confession. Now we'll focus on forgiveness for a few sessions. What does that mean? How will it happen? This is so scary. If Mary, Ruth, and Suzanne weren't with me, I couldn't do this. They have *power*, and they say they want to pray with me. How extraordinary that people can love this much.

Comment: *Confession* is an often-neglected part of the spiritual journey. It plays a central role in all religious healing rituals, primitive as well as Christian. The disclosure may be something related to sin, or it may be something the supplicant regards as shameful. Either way, the person doing the confessing feels bad about a past event or an attitude. He needs to confess this to someone in order to experience healing.

Those whose ministry focuses on love sometimes respond to a supplicant's confession by excusing him. They say things like "You were too young to know better," or "That wasn't a sin, it was just a mistake." Excusing someone's confession discounts the depths of his emotion and isolates him in his pain. He leaves ministry thinking that nobody understands him. His need to feel forgiven has not been met.

Confession is a healing experience because it is an emptying of one's self. An inner pain is exposed to someone, such as a friend, a loved one, a prayer team, or a priest in the sacrament of reconciliation. Ultimately, the confession is being made to God, but God as enfleshed in the Body of Christ. Ministers who truly hear and accept someone's confession allow the light of Christ to shine in the darkness. In the words of John:

> But if we live in light, as he is in light, we have a share in each other's life, and the blood of Jesus, his Son, cleanses us from all sin. . . . If we acknowledge our sins, he is trustworthy and upright, so that he will forgive our sins and will cleanse us from all evil (1 Jn 1:7, 9).

This scripture describes Dorothy's experience. She confessed to a prayer team what she had never been able to bring directly to God or to a priest. In so doing, she began the process of being cleansed from the wrong she had done.

Dorothy's October 15th journal entry reveals another aspect of the spirituality of a supplicant: She *believes the prayer team is able to help* her get well. ("They have *power.*") This raises her expectant trust (see Chapter 10). If Dorothy didn't believe the team could help her, she would discount their ministry. Prayer ministers are sometimes under-valued at large healing services that feature a renowned "healer." If at some point people are offered individual ministry at several locations throughout a room, a huge line will form in front of the "healer" while other ministers are nearly ignored. The audience's message in this case is clear: The superstar has magic. The other ministers don't.

Finally, Dorothy's October 15th entry shows she *realizes the team is willing to help* her get well. ("They say they want to pray with me.") She accurately links willingness with love. This heightens her level of trust in the team; she knows they will not harm her. Trust enables her to remove any protective shell she may have placed around herself. In so doing, she opens herself to God's healing touch.

Prayer Ministry: Spiritual Healing

After Dorothy's confession, Mary, Ruth and Suzanne realized that their goal in ministry was spiritual healing of the wound of abortion. They discerned the need for Dorothy to be reconciled with her aborted baby, with herself and with God (including, ultimately, the sacrament of reconciliation from a caring priest). With this in mind, the team devised a plan of action for the next phase of ministry.[4]

First, Dorothy became aware of her feelings about the abortion: guilt, pain, sorrow and anger at herself and at her boyfriend. The team accepted the appropriateness of each feeling. Doing this enabled Dorothy to see that Jesus did not want her to carry her twenty-year burden. She placed each feeling, one by one, at the foot of the cross. Slowly, relief began to replace oppression.

Next, ministry focused on the aborted baby. When Dorothy said she sensed it was a girl, the team asked her to choose a name for her. She chose Amelia. Using imagery prayer (see Chapter 6), Dorothy and the team brought Amelia to Jesus and asked him to baptize her.

A peak moment occurred when Dorothy mentally held Amelia in her arms and asked her forgiveness. Weeping profusely, she also asked Jesus for his forgiveness. The team anointed Dorothy with blessed oil and asked God to give her the gift of being able both to receive his forgiveness and to forgive herself. Finally, she handed Amelia to Jesus. Tenderly holding the baby in his arms, he assured Dorothy that she and Amelia would spend eternity together.

When they discerned she was ready, the team told Dorothy they thought the sacrament of reconciliation would bring added grace to her spiritual healing. Initially she resisted the idea, still worrying about the response she might encounter. Mary described the changes that had taken place since Dorothy had last received the sacrament, then wrote down the name of a compassionate "Rachel" priest. She explained that Rachel priests have been specially trained in ministry to people who are experiencing post-abortion trauma. She assured Dorothy that the mission of Rachel priests is to bring people back to God through forgiveness, not drive them away through condemnation. Dorothy said she felt torn between two feelings: a fear of facing a priest, but a longing to return to the sacraments. The team anointed her and asked God to give her the gift of courage.[5]

December 19: Oh Lord, this has been the wildest year of my life. On Monday I phoned the Rachel priest that Suzanne knows and asked if he could fit a half-hour appointment into his schedule. Secretly, I was praying he couldn't! But he could, so today I went and saw him. I was so nervous, I thought I'd throw up! But this Father Murphy seemed like such a gentle man that pretty soon I calmed down enough to tell him I wanted him to hear my confession.

When I told him it had been twenty years since my last confession, he said, "Welcome!" I said I'd forgotten how to go to confession, and he said to just tell him what was on my mind. It took me awhile to confess the abortion. I think I shed enough tears to flood us out of his office!

At the end of confession, Father Murphy told me that God loves me. God *loves* me! Oh, that feels so good. I've felt that love in prayer ministry, but today it's deeper. Today I feel like I've crawled into Jesus' lap, and he's rocking me. Lord, I want to stay here forever.

December 25: No eucharist has ever blessed me as much as today's did. Peace went through my whole body when I held the host in my hand. Just before, I was nervous because I'd never received communion in the hand before. But I decided that if I'd taken this many risks this year, I could take one more. Lord, what a *privilege* it is to receive you!

Tom and Jennifer were stunned when I got up and walked up front with them. They're amazed at how much I've changed. A few days ago I bought a new dress, my first in ages. When Jennifer saw it, she rushed into Tom's room and said, "Hey, Mom's got a new dress and it looks *good!*" Ah, the honesty of youth. I had to laugh. The sound of my laughter startled everyone, especially me. I'll bet it's been two years since I laughed.

December 31: On this day every year I look back over the past twelve months and see where I've been and where I'm going. Last December 31st was so bleak that I shudder to think of it. *This* December 31st, I feel like a new person, like some birth has taken place inside me. Colors look intense, music sounds crystal-clear, the smells of Christmas remind me of happy times when I was a child. It feels good to be *alive.*

A couple of days ago, Frank came home and said he had a belated Christmas present for us. He said it wasn't something you could wrap in paper, but still, it was a present. Then he said that secretly he'd been doing research for the past month and had discovered that there's a new, successful treatment for birthmarks! Jennifer shrieked, Tom said, "Cool!" I cried, Frank grinned, and Caitlin stared at us like we'd all lost our minds. Caitlin is going to be OK! The funny thing is, I've grown to love her as she is. Now, thanks to this wonderful Christmas present from God, soon I can take my baby out without needing to face people's cruelty.

Looking ahead to next year, I know that soon I'm going to leave prayer ministry. We talked about that in the last session. I said I was scared about trying to make it on my own. Suzanne said we're not *supposed* to make it on our own, people need each other to make it through life. The team said they're available if I want more ministry. Father Murphy said I'm welcome to return anytime, and I'll still go to my psychiatrist for a while (though I'm off the antidepressants). Then Mary told me that our parish is about to start a Bible study class. She thinks I'd get a lot out of it. I protested. My Bible is prehistoric, I told them, probably in the original language of Jesus' time. We laughed. Then Ruth wrote down the name of a modern Bible. They showed me how to look up scripture passages. "Just for practice," they had me look up one that they said fits me. It's about my "journey" over the past year and the fact that it won't be over as long as I'm here on earth. I have written it on a card and read it every time I think I already should have "arrived."

> I do not think of myself as having reached the finish line. I give no thought to what lies behind but push on to what is ahead. My entire attention is on the finish line as I run toward the prize to which God calls me — life on high in Christ Jesus (Phil 3:13–14, NAB).

Conclusion

This chapter's description of the rigors of the spiritual journey might lead ministers to conclude that no supplicant exists who possesses the needed traits, behaviors and attitudes for transformation into God's wholeness. This is true. Since no one reaches perfection in this life, it follows that every supplicant, and every minister, will be lacking in some areas of his being. Those imperfections will impact ministry, but they need not doom it.

Most people come to prayer ministry missing at least one of the traits needed for being a model supplicant. The more deeply wounded they are, the more lacking they are in a healthy spirituality. We ministers must resist the urge to lose heart when we encounter someone who, say, does not recognize his need for conversion. God always accepts us where we are and calls us forth from that point. In ministry we must do likewise.

The next two chapters of this book examine the spirituality of the supplicant from the prayer team's point of view. What is the enemy within each supplicant that must be conquered in order for ministry to succeed? (Chapter 9) And how can prayer teams help a supplicant move into greater faith in God, so as to open themselves up to the fullness of life? (Chapter 10) We use Dorothy's experiences to answer these questions.

Summary

The spirituality of the supplicant plays a key part in prayer ministry. Many traits, behaviors and attitudes help supplicants journey towards transformation into God's wholeness:

1. They recognize the need for conversion, the need to change in some way — behavior, attitudes, health, relationships.

2. They have enough motivation to take the strenuous journey towards wholeness.

3. They cooperate in their own healing and overcome the fear of loss of autonomy.

4. They trust God and the team not to harm them.

5. They are willing to experience heightened emotions.

6. They are open to receiving help from God through people, including the prayer team.

7. They have the ability to establish a committed relationship with the team.

8. They are willing to disclose information about themselves to the team, trusting the knowledge won't be abused.

9. They are willing to be active participants in their own healing, a process that includes every level of their being: physical, emotional, spiritual and relational.

10. They are willing to confess feelings to the team, emptying themselves of their inner pain so as to expose it to the healing light of Christ.

11. They believe the prayer team can help them.

12. They believe the prayer team is willing to help them.

Chapter Nine

The Enemy Within

What is the enemy within each
supplicant that needs to be conquered?

An invisible enemy lurked within Dorothy (Chapter 8). It couldn't be x-rayed or found in a blood test, but it was as real as a physical disease. It created a profound blackness that brought Dorothy to the brink of death. Mental health experts call the invisible enemy "demoralization." This chapter explores demoralization in depth because it is the greatest enemy to well-being that we face in ministering healing prayer. Whatever we can do to combat it will vastly improve a supplicant's growth toward wholeness.

Demoralization: What Is It?

Dr. Jerome Frank, a professor of psychiatry at Johns Hopkins University School of Medicine, studied all forms of healing in order to discover what they have in common. While analyzing the traits of *healing*, he began to perceive the traits of *illness*. He concluded that demoralization is the common factor in all illnesses:

> [Candidates for therapy of any kind] are conscious of having failed to meet their own expectations or those of others, or of being unable to cope with some pressing problem. They feel powerless to change the situation or themselves.... To various degrees the demoralized person feels isolated, hopeless, and helpless, and is preoccupied with merely trying to survive.[1]

In short, Dr. Frank concluded that:

Hopelessness + Helplessness + Isolation = Demoralization

135

Supplicants who seek prayer ministry vary in their severity of emotional, spiritual, or physical pain. Few are as immobilized as Dorothy. Typically they still function normally at work and sometimes at home. They smile and carry on social conversations when they need to, but their smiles veil an aching aloneness. They feel helpless because they have lost hope that they can cope with their hurts by themselves, using the resources available to them. Unless we are sensitized to their secret pain, the masks can fool us. We may not realize how cornered they feel.

Dorothy's initial state of mind portrayed demoralization's crippling traits. She felt physically trapped in her house with a baby whose birthmark provoked cruel comments. She felt her earlier abortion was an unforgivable sin that condemned her to hell. Her inability to tell anyone about the abortion left her in profound emotional isolation. Spiritually, she saw herself as a "hopeless case," helpless to change the past or the present. Worst of all, she could not imagine ever feeling better in the future. Dorothy was utterly demoralized.

Hopelessness vs. Hope

Everyday speech has reduced the word "hope" to mean a wish or desire, such as "I hope it doesn't rain tomorrow" or "I hope I get well." This use of hope reveals a half-hearted attitude towards healing. Used in its proper sense, hope is a strong word coming from a powerful mind set. It is difficult to attain, yet it plays a vital role in any kind of healing. And the lack of hope — hopelessness — plays an essential role in demoralization.

According to Jerome Frank,[2] *hopelessness is the inability to imagine a tolerable future.* Extreme hopelessness is even life-threatening. Examples of this can be found in nursing homes every day. Autopsies list no cause of death for some elderly residents, but loved ones often attest to a sudden loss of hope just prior to their death. People may say "Uncle Joe died of a broken heart," or "Aunt Susan just gave up." In reality, Uncle Joe and Aunt Susan became incapable of imagining a tolerable future. They died of hopelessness.

Our friend Iris is a eucharistic minister in a nursing home, and she tells the story of a patient named Myrtle, who lost her ability to walk when a flu kept her bedridden for several months. Myrtle's mind was fixed on one goal: relearning to walk. She lay in bed lifting her legs, stretching them and hounding aides to help her walk. After months of Myrtle's exercises and of Iris' prayers, the two of them convinced the staff to help. Initially she needed heavy support, then she learned to walk alone in a walker, then she learned to walk with a cane, then she left the nursing home and lived happily in an apartment — for ten years!

Myrtle's and Iris' paths crossed again when Myrtle broke her hip and ended up in the same nursing home. This time no amount of pleading would convince the staff to help her learn to walk again. They said it was a waste of time. Finally her physician sat down in her wheelchair, patted the arms of the chair, and said, "You've got to make up your mind. You are 93 years old. You are too old and weak; you will never walk again." With that, he left. Myrtle told Iris, "I'm going to die. There is no sense in living now." Within a week she was insane. Three weeks later she was dead, killed by a lethal dose of hopelessness.

Scientific experiments show that hope enters into the very fabric of life. Even animals show something akin to human hope and hopelessness.[3] Dr. Paul Pruyser, a specialist in the psychology of religion and a collaborator with Dr. Karl Menninger, was one of the early writers on the psychology of hope. He concluded that: "One little ray [of hope] is enough to invigorate some people. One moment of release from unbearable stress makes the world appear in a different image."[4]

In short, hope is an essential ingredient of life that encompasses the entire animal kingdom. Without hope, we perish. Myrtle died three weeks after her doctor ripped away all hope of her ever walking again. If people had not reached out to Dorothy, she would have died too. Her death certificate would have listed suicide as the cause of death, but the real reason would have come from an inability to imagine a tolerable future. The combination of receiving a prescription for medication plus starting psychiatric treatment gave her "one little ray of hope." As she said in her journal, "maybe pills will give me enough energy to do something around here." She felt invigorated just enough to see the world in a slightly different light.

Pruyser asserts that hope does not deny reality. Instead hope sees reality's wider scope, a scope that includes many unknowns. "This need not be a view of two worlds," he writes, "it is more likely to be two views of one world. . . . [Hoping] means surrender, not only to reality-up-to-now, but also to reality-from-now-on, including unknown novelties."[5]

Here Pruyser gets to the heart of hope as a Christian virtue. In times of trouble, reality-up-to-now means seeing ourselves trapped inescapably in our "problem." Reality-from-now-on means enlarging our view of things. It includes the notion that God sees us caught in our problem. *God* will help us, using infinite power and wisdom shaped by his love for us.

Hope-filled people see their desperate situation but refuse to believe this is all there is to reality. The virtue of hope says that God is dealing with life in ways that surpass our ability to grasp. *Hope, then, is a surrender, a "yes" to faith in God's existence, wisdom, power and, most of all, his love.* God invites us to say yes to an unimaginable future in which the only guarantee is that he will be with us. This is quite a surrender for any person.

Scripture overflows with stories of the yeses of holy people. Mary's "yes" at the time of the Annunciation enabled the Son of God to enter the world. Jesus' "yes" in the Garden of Gethsemane has blessed creation for all eternity. Scripture also includes stories of people's "no"s. As recounted in Genesis, humankind's first sin was succumbing to the desire to "be like gods" (Gn 3:5). We've been re-peating the same mistake ever since. Instead of hoping in the Lord, saying "yes" to him, the constant temptation exists to seize control of our own destiny.

Sometimes, we who profess belief in God even try to control him! We know we cannot make God our servant, but perhaps we can manipulate him as a child would a parent. Maybe, we reason, we can please God with religious practices or acts of self-denial. Our holiness will so impress God that he'll feel compelled to shower a good job or great vacation weather down upon us. Jesus did not display this attitude. Even when he was in agony, he prayed with hope, not manipulation: "Father . . . if you are willing, take this cup away from me. Nevertheless, let your will be done, not mine" (Lk 22:42). Jesus surrendered to a Father's love that knew the unimaginable glory that lay beyond the crucifixion.

Manipulation denies the mystery of God's love, yet ministers and supplicants usually bring some of these attitudes into the ministry of religious healing. Jan recalls a workshop whose purpose was to teach people how to "claim God's promises." Pointing out passages of promises in scripture, the instructor said if the students combined these texts and laid them before the Lord, he'd do what was asked because he had promised. The implication was that if God didn't respond, the right formula hadn't been found.

Manipulation is *not* surrender to the Lord's presence in an unimaginable future, which lies at the heart of the virtue of hope. People in control don't *need* hope. They may think that getting God to do something is the same as hoping in him, but they're mistaken. It's only when someone experiences herself as being a cherished child of a loving God that she realizes she does not need to control her destiny. God's love is unfailing, and in surrendering to him, something good always happens.

This is hard to believe. We all have had many experiences of "bad things" happening to us, events that seem to point to a powerful God who is at best capricious and at worst vengeful. The ministry of religious healing builds upon a healed image of a God that we can truly hope in. We worship one whom we need not cajole, plead or bargain with. Our God knows our needs before we mention them or even know them ourselves. In non-controlling prayer ministry the words of Jesus come to life:

> That is why I am telling you not to worry about your life and what you are to eat, nor about your body and what you are to wear.... Your heavenly Father knows you need them all. Set your hearts on his kingdom first, and on God's saving justice, and all these other things will be given you as well (Mt 6:25, 32b–33).

Surrender is *not* the passivity of fatalism, an attitude that says "There is nothing that I can do, so just let happen what is going to happen." Instead, yielding to God requires action, both by ministers and supplicants. Jesus modeled supplicant activity for us by involving the sick in their own healing. Even Lazarus needed to walk out of the tomb, wrappings and all, when Jesus raised him from the dead (Jn 11:43–44).

Saying yes to the will of God calls for great activity on our part, but it flows from humility. God is in control, and one dimension of that control is the fact that he acts *through* us. Liberation from an "inescapable" situation is indeed given but it must be actively received. We must use what has been given. Neither the minister nor the supplicant is a puppet dangling from strings held in God's hands.

Dorothy discovered that hope is hard work. Popping antidepressants would have been easy. Taking a lethal dose of sleeping pills would have been easier still. That one action would have made her master of her own destiny, in charge of the outcome of her "inescapable" situation. Instead, she chose the longer, more difficult journey out of hopelessness, leaving the results up to God's wisdom, power and love. Letting God be God meant facing long-buried feelings and revealing her abortion to the prayer team. It meant giving up being the center of her own universe. Slowly she became able look beyond herself to God and to people.

Whenever a team prays with a supplicant, it faces the challenge of active surrendering. This takes time! Dorothy's healing occurred over a period of many months. Much of her healing involved a progressive giving of her life to God. A peak moment of surrender took place when she risked telling the team about her abortion. Another key moment came when she sought to be reunited with God through the sacrament of reconciliation.

Teams often yearn for more "spiritual power" in order to make the supplicant "have faith." They may fantasize that if they could do one *big* prayer, she would be healed instantly. Lacking this quick, magic power, they may feel overcome with feelings of hopelessness, deciding their supplicant is too difficult. When tempted to give up, teams need to pray for an increase of hope, both for the supplicant and for themselves.

Ultimately the Christian virtue of hope is possible only in the context of a relationship with God, a relationship that is mediated by Christ as he is today, the Body of Christ. In other words, Christian hope occurs by being in relationship with God through other Christians, including ministers of healing. We can wish or long for something in isolation from any one else, but we cannot *hope* for it in complete isolation from others. *Hope is given by the Holy Spirit, mediated by the Body of Christ, and received by the individual.*

Helplessness

Hopelessness is the key ingredient in demoralization, but it implies the other two: helplessness and isolation. We are hopeless because we are helpless, that is, *helplessness is the feeling of being caught in an inescapable situation.* We believe the situation is inescapable because, alone, we do not have the resources to escape.

We are isolated from those who can help free us. Hope and help are as intertwined as partners in a marriage; you cannot think of hope without thinking of help, and help implies some resource outside ourselves which will enable us to escape from the inescapable.

American culture promotes the idea that hope is self-generated, and needing help is shameful. This lie says the "truly strong" never need help. It denies the reality of humanity's interdependency on one another. Educator and journalist Father W. F. Lynch says:

> [This fantasy] will make more people sick and sick people sicker still if not qualified. . . . Hope is truly on the inside of us, but hope is an interior sense that there is help on the outside of us. There are times when we are especially aware that our own purely inward resources are not enough, that they have to be added to from the outside. . . . This need of help is a . . . continuing fact for each human being.[6]

Dorothy knew that her "inward resources" were depleted. Her problem was she didn't know how to find help outside herself. Fortunately, caring people came and *offered* her help. Husband, psychiatrist, neighbor, prayer team — all these people reached out to show that external help was available. Once they relieved her feelings of helplessness, hope began to blossom.

When Dorothy was in the depths of her depression, telling her "have hope" would have been futile. This hollow phrase is often the way people try to help a demoralized person. Writer William Styron encountered these people when he was wrestling with a profound depression. Later he wrote that "calling 'chin up!' from the safety of the shore to a drowning person is tantamount to insult."[7] People who use phony cheer leave the supplicant feeling *more* demoralized because they emotionally distance themselves from the sufferer. Her pain is not their pain; they can leave the scene, free and deluded into thinking they have "helped."

Each person who comes to us for help has reached the awareness that their inner resources are not enough. Most of them have some expectation that we can help, or else they would not have sought out prayer ministry. We must demonstrate that our ministry is capable of supplying that needed resource. Words are not enough. Supplicants must *experience* our help. (Chapter 10 describes how to do this.)

Isolation

The third element of demoralization is isolation. Basically the cure for isolation lies in the power of community, a subject which we cover in Chapter 5. In team ministry, a group of people lovingly enters into the alienating world of illness with the supplicant. Their response of hope and offer of help is a powerful means of combating isolation.

Faith

In religious healing, faith — as in faith healing — often means a naive confidence in another human's power to heal. Sometimes it means faith in results, i.e., in getting better. In short, "faith" often takes on a false meaning.

Even without distortions, faith carries meanings that do not apply to healing. The Apostles' Creed binds diverse Christian denominations together: "I believe in God, the Father Almighty" is creedal faith, a confession of belief in God's existence and in the basic tenets of our religion. It does not address the faith we think of when we talk about healing. Anglican priest Leslie D. Weatherhead discusses many of faith's biblical and theological meanings in his book *Psychology, Religion and Healing*.[8] He defines Christian faith as: "the response of the whole man, thinking, feeling and willing, to the impact of God in Christ, by which man comes into a conscious personal relationship with God."

So the essence of Christian faith is a relationship with God. Without that, we are left with a hollow, intellectual assent to God's being: "You believe in the one God — that is creditable enough, but even the demons have the same belief, and they tremble with fear" (Jas 2:19).

Later Weatherhead adds to his definition of Christian faith:

> Christian faith is faith in a person. . . . It is our maximum response to God in Christ. . . , a personal relationship with a living friend by faith. . . . The Christian is to have faith in Christ because he is Christ, and that faith means "following" whether healing is gained or not.[9]

This statement begins to link our relationship with God with faith as regards healing. Weatherhead writes:

The faith required for healing is not, and never has been, theological in its character. That is to say it has not been a faith
in the truth of creedal statements. It has rather been *expectant
trust* in a person.[10]

In other words: *faith (as regards healing) is expectant trust in
God.* Religious healing focuses on a person (Christ), *not* on a result.
Jesus remarked on this type of faith when he cured the centurion's
servant (Mt 8:5–13). When the centurion said, "Sir, I am not worthy
to have you under my roof; just give the word and my servant will
be cured," his focus was on Jesus, *not* on the curing of a disease.
The centurion placed his trust in a person: "I am under authority
myself . . . ."

A footnote in the *New Jerusalem Bible* elaborates:

The faith that Jesus asks for from the outset of his public life
and throughout his subsequent career, is that act of trust and
of self-abandonment by which people no longer rely on their
own strength and policies but commit themselves to the power
and guiding word of him in whom they believe. Jesus asks for
this faith especially when he works his miracles . . . . Since faith
demands the sacrifice of the whole person, mind and heart, it is
not an easy act of humility to perform; many decline it . . . (Mt
8, footnote b).

The centurion abandoned himself to Jesus' authority in the servant's illness, even without Jesus coming to his home. The gospel
writer records, "When Jesus heard this he was astonished and said
to those following him, 'In truth I tell you, in no one in Israel have
I found faith (expectant trust) as great as this'" (Mt 8:10).

When people focus on results (cures) instead of on a person
(Jesus), the results can be disastrous:

One of the damning indictments of some healing missions is that
the onus is always on the patient. If he is healed, he is praised
for his "faith." If he is unhealed, it is implied that he had no
faith. The mission spreads a false conception about the nature
of faith, the purpose of religion and the problem of suffering.
Very great harm is done both by the successes and the failures
of such a mission.[11]

Ria is a woman who was harmed in ways that Weatherhead notes.
A broken collar bone left her with limited mobility of her right arm,

so a church prayer group prayed eagerly for her. Several people prophesied that she would be completely healed and exhorted her to claim her healing. Having noted no improvement during the next week, Ria asked the group to pray again. They did so, this time with a noticeable lack of fervor. A week later, with still no improvement, Ria did not have the courage to ask for prayer again. But the prayer group leader approached her, questioned her, then scolded her for her lack of "faith." He admonished Ria to confess her sin of faithlessness and claim in full confidence the healing that the Lord had promised her. Ria burst into tears and never returned to that church.

When "faith healing" doesn't help people like Ria, they decide they either lack the "faith" to be healed, or else have unconfessed sins. From this it is a short leap to conclude that not even God can (or more accurately, will) help them. Forceful, power-centered ministry leaves people feeling more hopeless, helpless and isolated than if they had had no ministry at all.

The man at the Pool of Bethesda would have understood this problem. He lay beside the pool, where

> crowds of sick people — blind, lame, paralysed — waited for the water to move; for at intervals the angel of the Lord came down into the pool, and the water was disturbed, and the first person to enter the water after this disturbance was cured of any ailment he suffered from (Jn 5:3–4, *JB*).

When Jesus approached and said "Do you want to be well again?" a litany of demoralization poured forth that echoes through every age. "'Sir,' replied the sick man, 'I have no one (*isolation*) to put me into the pool when the water is disturbed; and while I am still on the way, someone else gets down there before me (*helplessness*)'" (Jn 5:7). Isolation and helplessness point to the situation's *hopelessness*.

Jesus' loving presence must have reduced the sick man's feelings of isolation and given him a ray of hope that here, at last, was the help for which he'd been waiting for thirty-eight years. Today countless people lie at twentieth-century Bethesdas, longing for the Body of Christ to bring Jesus to them so that they can physically, emotionally and spiritually walk again. Let us pray for ears to hear the desperation that is wrapped in silence.

Summary

Demoralization is the greatest enemy to well-being that we face in ministering healing prayer.

Demoralization = hopelessness + helplessness + isolation.

Hope: (1) surrenders to reality-up-to-now; (2) says yes to faith in God's wisdom, power and love; (3) actively says yes to an unimaginable future in which the only guarantee is God's loving presence; (4) gives up the desire for self-sufficiency; gives up insisting on knowing all; (5) gives up being in control and instead hands control over to God; (6) gives up being the center of one's own universe; (7) gives up the right to determine the outcome of a current problem; (8) is only possible in the context of a relationship with God; (9) is a virtue which is given by the Holy Spirit, mediated by the Body of Christ, and received by the individual.

Helplessness: the feeling of being caught in an inescapable situation. A major task of prayer ministers is to supply outside help to the supplicant.

Isolation: In team ministry, a group of people lovingly enters into the alienating world of illness with the supplicant. Their response of hope and offer of help combat isolation.

Faith (as regards healing):   expectant trust in God. It focuses on a person (Christ), *not* on a result (cures).

Chapter Ten

"Help My Lack of Trust!"

How can ministers of pastoral care help
conquer a supplicant's hidden enemy?

> [The boy's father said], "If out of the kindness of your heart you
> can do anything to help us, please do!" Jesus said, "'If you can'?
> Everything is possible to a man who trusts." The boy's father
> immediately exclaimed, "I do believe! Help my lack of trust!"
> (Mk 9:22b–24, *NAB*).

Here, the possessed boy's father spoke for millions of people
who *do* believe in Jesus' power to heal but need help from the Body
of Christ to raise their expectant trust about their own healing. Jesus
used all the resources available to him to combat the intense demoralization he found in the hurting people of his day. To the extent
that we do likewise in our ministry, our supplicants will experience
healing. Raising expectant trust is *our* job, not the supplicant's:

> It is the church's duty to call out [expectant trust] in all the
> healthy ways known to her. If this were done, we have every
> reason to believe that many who are sick would be healed.[1]

This chapter describes how ministers can help people who lack
the trust ("faith," as some people call it) to be healed. It is a contin-
uation of Chapters 8 and 9, in which we reflected on Dorothy's story
of depression, demoralization and experience of ministry. Here we
discuss seven ways to raise expectant trust. These techniques are effective ways to combat hopelessness, helplessness and isolation, the
three key ingredients in demoralization (discussed in Chapter 8).

1. Convey the Prospect of Help

Before Dorothy could find relief from her depression, she needed to know that help was available to her. She also needed to be *motivated* to use that help. Her husband, Frank, told her a psychiatrist could help, found a competent one for her, then urged her to attend at least several sessions. Her neighbor, Judy, broached the subject of a prayer team, said she thought they could help her feel better, then offered to accompany her to her first session. Finally, Suzanne, the telephone contact person, reassured Dorothy about the prayer ministry process and told her how much relief people experience through ministry.

Together, Frank, Judy and Suzanne conveyed the prospect of help to Dorothy. They did this, first, in the context of their rapport with her. Their connectedness with her relieved some of her profound isolation. They took Dorothy into their hearts through unconditional, non-judgmental love. Their respect for her left her free to decide whether or not she would use the help of prayer ministry. This gave her a small sense of power and autonomy, which helped counteract her feelings of helplessness. Their sensitivity to Dorothy's struggle to admit the need for help left her dignity intact.[2]

So even before she started prayer ministry, a glimmer of hope had appeared on Dorothy's horizon, a message that all was not lost. She had been given enough information to know what she could expect prayer ministry to be like and what was expected of her. She knew that Frank, Judy and Suzanne all were willing to help her begin the process of healing. This raised her expectant trust that something good was going to happen through the outside help she was about to receive.

Most of us have experienced relief from pain just by, say, making a doctor's appointment or walking into his office for a visit. No words have been spoken, no medicine swallowed, yet as if by magic, we begin to feel a bit better. Knowing that help is available raises our expectant trust. At that moment, we begin to get well.

2. Get Supplicant to "Tell His/Her Story"

Dorothy spent half of her first ministry session simply telling her story. The team made this possible, first, by explaining the process of ministry in order to alleviate her anxiety, then by using empathetic statements when she was overcome by emotion, and finally by being attentive listeners. By the end of two sessions, Dorothy discovered that even when she told the team "bad things," they still loved her. She wrote in her journal that "the team didn't faint" when she said she couldn't feel love for her disfigured baby. The ministers reacted to her disclosure with Christ-like, unconditional love.

Enabling supplicants to tell their story combats demoralization because it removes isolation and relieves their loneliness. Furthermore, when supplicants reveal their inner self to caring ministers, they allow the light of Christ to shine into the confusion of their feelings. This, in turn, mobilizes their expectancy that help *is* forthcoming — from God, from others and from themselves.

Telling their story helps supplicants name previously unnamed facts, wounds or feelings. And putting a name on something is the first step towards bringing it under control. As mentioned in Chapter 8, Alcoholics Anonymous uses this method to combat the profound demoralization that alcoholics experience.

In prayer ministry, getting a supplicant to tell her story is an unfolding, ongoing event. It took Dorothy several months to muster the courage to tell the team about her abortion. What started as a story about external problems (Caitlin) and current wounds (the public's response to Caitlin's birthmark) evolved into a story about internal struggles (self-condemnation) and past wounds (the abortion). The unfolding nature of telling one's story underscores the fact that ministry is a dynamic process. We ministers of religious healing never reach the point of having figured someone out. Surprises await us at every session as a supplicant tells us about her life and her deepest self. We must treat these stories as sacred revelation.

3. Demonstrate Help

When Dorothy brought Caitlin to ministry, the team's spontaneous delight at seeing Caitlin showed Dorothy that this was a baby, not a birthmark with a pulse. Their display of love and joy helped Dorothy begin to love her child. This showed her that she now could do what she was unable to do prior to ministry. She could love her baby. Dorothy *experienced* the team's ability to help. Because this event happened during the course of healing ministry, it increased her expectancy of more help being forthcoming through the team for her other problems.

Supplicants need to know that our ministry can help in the healing of their wounds. When we demonstrate that we can supply external help to them, their feelings of helplessness subside. Help *is* available from an outside source — us. The lived, felt experience of our help raises their expectant trust.

4. Heighten Emotions

The use of heightened emotions has been so abused by healing ministers in the public media that many people discount its role in healing. They equate it with unrestrained emotionalism. For instance, a "faith healer" works a crowd by crying or shouting mass suggestion ("I sense the Lord is healing someone *right now* of cancer") and outright orders ("Get up from your wheelchair!") This is a misuse of heightened emotion, a blatant manipulation which violates the sacredness of people's feelings, souls and journeys with God.

Used correctly, heightened emotion means responding appropriately to something wonderful or painful or holy or evil. It means a genuineness in ministry that gives supplicants permission to experience *all* their emotions — positive and negative. Many people never have received this permission before they experience it in ministry.

Prior to starting ministry, Dorothy had suffocated her emotions of guilt and self-condemnation beneath a blanket of depression. The depression began to lift when her prayer team saw Caitlin and responded with genuine joy. They oohed and aahed as most people do when they see a baby, and their own emotions of joy enabled Dorothy to see her child with new eyes — eyes of love. Her newly aroused feelings of love caused her to weep for joy, and the team responded to her tears by first holding her and Caitlin and then anointing them for bonding with each other.

Teams need to discover ways to help supplicants experience heightened emotions *without* violating their minds and souls. Creating a worship experience (Chapter 4) is one of the most effective ways to achieve this goal. Setting up a sacred space, playing soothing music, reading scripture passages that directly relate to a supplicant's need, all these create an environment in which he can experience the full range of his emotions, joy, pain, sorrow, fear, anger, love. The team's genuineness and love can convey the message that these heightened emotions are God-given and acceptable. This removes the isolation of the feelings and opens the supplicant up to the healing touch of God.

5. Use Sacramentals

Jesus often used physical items (sacramentals) to raise the expectant trust of the sick. For instance, in Jn 9:6–7, when a blind man came to him seeking healing, he made a paste out of dirt and saliva, put the paste (one sacramental) on the man's eyes, then told him to go wash in the pool of Siloam (another sacramental). These items did not possess magical qualities. Instead, these were the physical elements, the sacramentals, that Jesus used in order to raise the blind man's expectancy that healing was in the process of taking place. (Chapter 11 explores the difference between magic and sacramentals.)

Dorothy's prayer team used blessed oil to anoint her and Caitlin for bonding with one another. The oil added a physical aspect to an emotional healing that was occurring between mother and child. It helped arouse Dorothy's expectant trust that bonding was, indeed, taking place.

Sacramentals are physical symbols of God's loving care and of his power to heal. People need these symbols because life occurs on more than a misty, spiritual plane. It also takes place on physical, emotional and relational levels. A team's belief in the power of sacramentals and the way they communicate that belief has a bearing on a supplicant's expectant trust. Used well (i.e., not as magic, but as holy symbols) sacramentals lift supplicants out of their feelings of hopelessness. God is *present* in ministry, and the experience of that truth heals.[3]

6. Instruct Supplicants

Lots of instructing goes on in good ministry, but not in the form of a lecture. Instead, instructing in ministry comes in many shapes with a single purpose: to change a supplicant's wounded view of reality. These words of Jesus reflect our goal in instructing: "You will come to know the truth, and the truth will set you free" (Jn 8:32).

Exposing and refuting lies is one form of instructing. Dorothy believed that some sins (e.g., her abortion) were unforgivable. Therefore she thought she was damned to hell, no matter how strongly she yearned for reconciliation with God. The team exposed that belief as being untrue. They refuted the lie, first through the use of scripture, then through referring her to a compassionate priest who could administer the sacrament of reconciliation. Their instructing liberated Dorothy from her feelings of hopelessness and self-condemnation.

Giving information at a teachable moment is another form of instructing. When Dorothy first came to ministry, she was ready only for unconditional love. The team needed to wait for the right time, the teachable moment in her spiritual journey, before they gave her information about, for example, the new rite of the sacrament of reconciliation.

Discernment is crucial with this type of instructing! It's easy to haul out important information at the wrong moment and present it to a supplicant who cannot yet receive it. Like trying to teach calculus to a first-grader, the effort fails. This leaves everyone feeling bad — ministers are discouraged and supplicants feel guilty, overwhelmed, or hostile.

Still another form of instructing is *helping supplicants locate and use other resources of help.* Dorothy had never read the Bible before she came to ministry. The team needed to lead her through a step-by-step process to teach her how to use this life-giving resource. First they wrote out a scripture verse for her on a card; then after awhile they showed her how to look up verses herself; then finally they referred her to a scripture study group so that her faith could continue to grow. By the time Dorothy left ministry, the team had given her a life-long treasure: the word of God.

One final form of instructing is *correcting unrealistic expectations.* In Dorothy's final journal entry, she said she'd told the team she was afraid to end ministry because, "I was scared about trying to make it on my own." She thought that if she were normal, she should be able to continue her spiritual and emotional journey with no help from anyone. Suzanne countered this expectation with the statement that "people need each other in order to make it through life." She pointed out that Dorothy would still be continuing with her psychiatrist. The team said they were available for follow-up ministry if it was needed, and Father Murphy had invited her to return to see him whenever she wanted. Correcting Dorothy's unrealistic expectations kept her from sinking back into isolation.

Most supplicants' expectations are subtle and unspoken. Rarely are they as dramatic as someone coming for ministry and announcing, "By the end of this session, I'm going to be able to walk again!" Therefore, ministers need to be good listeners.

7. Help Supplicants Recognize Changes That Take Place

We believe that something good *always* happens in good ministry. The challenge is for everyone to see that good and praise God for it. No difficulty would exist if supplicants always received precisely what they asked us to pray for. If everyone that sought a particular healing experienced it by the end of a ministry session, we ministers would be little more than spiritual vending machines. People would come to us, select the healing they wanted, press our buttons and — voila! — they would get what they asked for.

The good news is that we are not spiritual machines. That's also the bad news because it means looking beyond the obvious to find *all* the healings that occur. They may be big or little; spiritual, emotional, physical or relational; asked for or not asked for. "And now, I make all things new" (Rv 21:5, *TEV*) invites us to *see* what things God makes new in ministry. We must discern those changes, then help our supplicants to see them too.

Discernment of results rarely happens without a plan for ministry. The plan starts with a long range goal, e.g., the healing of Dorothy's depression. But reaching that goal usually means adopting and implementing short range, well defined goals, e.g., bonding Dorothy with Caitlin, praying with her about her aborted baby. Implementing our plans removes a key component in demoralization, helplessness, because something is being *done*. And because it's being done with a team, it also removes isolation. External help is visible, tangible, and audible.

The expression "nothing succeeds like success" holds true in healing ministry as much as in the rest of life. After adopting and implementing our plans for ministry, we must evaluate its results to discover where it has been a success. Recognizing healing that already has taken place increases a supplicant's expectancy that further healing will occur. And since changes have been noticed and discussed in the context of ministry, they are seen as the result of ministry. The supplicant comes to believe that the changes have occurred as the result of God's loving, personal action.

Often we need to help supplicants recognize changes that take place, especially if those changes are subtle or unexpected. Then we need to offer praise and thanksgiving to God. This points to the source of the healing and keeps it clear that *we* are not that source. It helps supplicants believe that God has *personally* touched them. This, in turn, gives them an experience of hope in its most profound meaning. This hope increases people's trust in the Lord and opens them to the fullness of life that God offers them.

Cautions About Raising Expectant Trust

We walk a tightrope when we strive to raise our supplicants' expectant trust. It's easy to fall to one side or the other as we promise them everything or nothing. For centuries the church erred toward the "nothing" side by urging people to "offer up" their suffering — their pain was "God's will."[4]

Now some ministers of religious healing are leaning toward the "everything" side of the tightrope. In the absence of discernment, they assure people that God will answer their specific prayers in a specific way at a specific time. Often scripture passages are used to convey their message. When the promised result fails to materialize, it causes *more* demoralization, not less. Hope is dashed, faith is shattered, trust is broken. Supplicants leave ministry in worse shape than when they arrived, because now they believe not even God can heal them.

It takes spiritual maturity and discipline to resist the temptation to make hollow promises. In the presence of suffering, words like "everything will be OK" automatically rise to our lips. Such empty reassurances ignore the fact that what is possible in theory may not be possible in reality. Prayer teams may lack the time a supplicant needs for extensive ministry. Supplicants may live in surroundings that counteract God's healing power. Factors like these should give us pause before we bypass discernment in our rush to relieve someone's suffering.

Discerning Results

Sometimes at the end of ministry a supplicant reports that "nothing happened." In our experience, seldom does *nothing* happen, but supplicants often have unrealistic or narrow expectations about ministry. These can block the very healing that's being sought. For instance, if Dorothy had arrived at her first ministry session expecting her depression to totally vanish in one hour, she indeed would have felt that "nothing happened" during that hour. Her mind would have been so focused on that one goal that she would have been unable to receive God's unconditional love offered to her through the team. She would have left ministry more depressed than when she arrived.

When a supplicant reports that nothing happened during ministry, this gives the team the opportunity to help him clarify his expectations and identify changes that have taken place but escaped his notice. Was he expecting instant results? Was he seeking only physical healing? Was his mind set on a particular *way* to experience God, say, through "warm and fuzzy" feelings? All these expectations can blind him to God's broader vision for his journey towards wholeness, a journey that is filled with surprises and unforeseen turns.

Sometimes, even after careful investigation, everyone concludes that, indeed, no change has taken place. If the team accepts this fact as readily as it accepts positive results, it avoids the triple traps of blame, despair and demoralization. Freely acknowledging no results allows everyone to ask the obvious question of why and to seek the answer through prayer. Praying for discernment can deepen a team's understanding of how to minister to this supplicant in this situation at this time. And clearer discernment increases the hope of a successful outcome in ministry. As with the rest of life, the path towards victory often passes through a few valleys of failure.

Conclusion

Like food that feeds the body, expectant trust usually comes to people from outside themselves. It is not self-generated. Instead, it is a power that the Body of Christ possesses and must offer to those who are demoralized. If we ministers of religious healing expect our supplicants to magically "have faith," they will depart unhealed and more wounded than when they arrived. Raising expectant trust is *our* job. It is one of the most important tasks in our ministry. Jesus recognized that fact in his ministry to the wounded of his day. When we carry on his mission, we too must do all we can to "help the lack of trust" that burdens our supplicants.

Summary

This chapter describes how ministers can help people who lack the trust ("faith") to be healed. It discusses seven ways to raise expectant trust:

1. Convey the prospect of help.
2. Get supplicants to "tell their story."
3. Demonstrate help.
4. Heighten emotions.
5. Use sacramentals.
6. Instruct supplicants. This includes:
   a. exposing and refuting lies,
   b. giving information at a teachable moment,
   c. helping supplicants locate and use other resources of help,
   d. correcting unrealistic expectations.
7. Help supplicants recognize changes that take place.

In striving to raise expectant trust, ministers of religious healing should avoid making hollow promises because these will *increase* a supplicant's demoralization, not relieve it.

Discerning results enables supplicants to clarify their expectations and identify changes that have taken place. As teams help in this process, supplicants come to believe (to "have faith," to trust in God) that the healing they've experienced will continue.

Chapter Eleven

The Problem of Miracles

*Why does the issue of miracles keep
healing ministry out of parishes?*

Religion gets into trouble whenever it falls in love with the spectacular. Thousands flock to see the face of Christ on a church wall, while they miss seeing his face in a hurting neighbor. Hundreds of thousands pour over the newest book that predicts the world is coming to an end next month, while they forget to serve God this month. Desperate people stampede a "healer" who has just come to town.

Miracles are the sensational side of religious healing, and those who make them a central focus of their ministry have created havoc for all ministers of religious healing. The obsession with miracles takes people's eyes off of God and puts them onto results (miracles) and "healers" (those who *make* miracles happen). This generates a circus atmosphere instead of peace, order, and worship. Worse yet, supplicants who don't experience a miraculous healing often feel guilty for having somehow failed.

The sensational easily moves into fraud. Sometimes the deceit is for personal gain, but often the deceiver simply wants to give people an exciting experience of God. The Acts of the Apostles describes Simon the Magician's abuse of charisms:

> When Simon saw that the Spirit was given through the laying on
> of the apostles' hands, he offered them money, with the words,
> "Give me the same power so that anyone I lay my hands on will
> receive the Holy Spirit" (Acts 8:18–19).

Peter said, "May you and your money rot — thinking that God's gift can be bought!" He went on to point out the root of Simon's problem, and the root of today's problem with miracles: "Your heart is not steadfastly set on God" (Acts 8:20, 21b, *NAB*).

When our hearts are not "steadfastly set on God," our ministry will fail in its mission to help people move forward on their spiritual journey. Focusing on miracles instead of on God may bring short term, dramatic results, but in the long run it discredits ministry in the eyes of the public and of church authorities. This, in turn, keeps healing out of parishes because it scares people. If we want to bring healing back into our faith communities, where it existed in the early church, then we must see miracles in a new light.

Miracles: The Popular View

Ask 100 people what a miracle is and all 100 of them probably will say something to the effect that it is an event that defies the laws of nature. It cannot be explained by what scientists now know. Ask for an example of a miracle, and people often think of physical healings: Jesus raising Lazarus from the dead or, today, someone's sudden, complete remission from cancer.

The popular definition of a miracle divides the world into opposing parts: physical vs. spiritual, profane vs. sacred, natural vs. supernatural. In this approach, God normally is absent in the physical, natural order. He is "out there" where we cannot reach him except through prayer. In response to those prayers, God occasionally rouses himself, comes down to earth, and "does" a miracle.

When the world is divided into opposing parts like this, people feel pressured to choose which side they're on — do they, or do they not, believe in miracles?[1] Some give an unequivocal yes to this question, while others handle the issue by ignoring it. Others take a more sophisticated approach and explain away all events that appear to defy the laws of nature. They believe that the New Testament descriptions of miracles were a way to convey deep truths to an uneducated society, e.g., the healing of the man born blind was a healing of spiritual, not physical, blindness; Jesus' resurrection was spiritual, not physical; the virgin birth was not literal.

In a divided, natural vs. supernatural world, the scientific response is to deny or discount the existence of the supernatural. The scientist says she cannot find God by using empirical methods. Therefore, God does not exist, and neither do miracles. Faced with a mysterious event, the scientific skeptic says that everything can be explained via the laws of nature: we just don't know those laws well enough yet.

Some people straddle both sides of the issue by admitting that miracles used to exist because the early church needed God's direct help, but now the world has outgrown the need. Like a child that now can cross the street without a grownup holding her hand, we now can live our lives without God's intervention. This approach puts God into the category of a creator who started things off right and then told us to carry on from there.

In the end, the varied responses to the popular view of miracles all fall short. Some responses deny the existence of God. Some pit him against the very world he created. Other responses make the creator subservient to the laws of nature, and still others arise from a theology of human independence from God. Perhaps the problem does not lie with these responses. Instead, the problem arises from the popular answer to the question: What are miracles?

The Catholic church teaches that miracles do exist, that Jesus performed them and that they have value. Many Protestant churches teach likewise. Unfortunately, theologians never have been able to agree upon a single definition of "miracle."[2] A miracle brings us face to face with one of the mysteries of our faith. These mysteries cannot be fully understood, but they must be explored. Otherwise, our spiritual journey would grind to a halt. What follows is an expanded view of miracles that takes us beyond the popular view, keeps us from idolizing the sensational, and allows us to keep our hearts "steadfastly set on God."

Miracles: An Expanded View

Today, theologians are beginning to move away from the *what* and *how* of miracles to the question of *why*. Typically an expanded view of miracles includes four elements:[3]

1. Transcendence, i.e., some observable, extraordinary event. The key word here is "extraordinary." Traditionally, the transcendence has been physical. Jesus walking on water fits the idea of physical transcendence.

Limiting the definition of miracles to the physical realm can blind us to other observable, extraordinary events. For instance, Pentecost found the disciples secluded in an upper room in Jerusalem.

But after the descent of the Holy Spirit, they suddenly became fearless proclaimers of the good news. Something happened that visibly transformed them from quivering survivors into bold messengers. We believe that emotional and spiritual transcendence can fit the definition of miracles as much as physical transcendence.[4]

2. *A religious context in which the extraordinary event occurs.* Amazing events happen every day, but unless they happen within a religious context, people don't call them miracles. Luke's description of a catch of fish (Lk 5:1–11) is recognized as miraculous because it takes place in a religious context. Jesus used Simon Peter's fishing boat as a site for teaching a crowd on shore about the word of God. Then he told the fishermen to lower their nets, and a huge quantity of fish was brought into the same boat from which, moments earlier, Jesus had been preaching the word of God. And right after the catch, Jesus invited Peter and his companions to follow him.

3. *Sign value, i.e., the event points to God.*   An event that points to God reveals his presence, power, care and concern for us. It reveals what God is like and speaks a message from him through the action, saying in effect, "I am with you. I love you and am calling you close to me."

The event that has sign value is external and visible. For instance, the miraculous catch of fish pointed to the fact that Jesus was Lord of nature. Also, it showed Peter that God had entered his life, and was calling him to be a disciple of Jesus. This realization frightened him:

> When Simon Peter saw this he fell at the knees of Jesus saying, "Leave me, Lord; I am a sinful man." For he and all his companions were completely awestruck at the catch they had made; so also were James and John, sons of Zebedee, who were Simon's partners. But Jesus said to Simon, "Do not be afraid; from now on it is people you will be catching" (Lk 5:8–10).

4. *A moral disposition in the observer.*   People must be open to religious truth in order to see an event's transcendent meaning. Without that openness, they can witness extraordinary phenomena and say, "Miracles? What miracles?" Or they explain them away as a sign of something other than God. A lack of faith, a lack of good will or a terror of the spiritual blinds them as surely as someone in a cave whose light has gone out. The truth lies before them, but they cannot, or will not, see it.

Jesus often encountered this problem in his ministry. For example, when he cured a blind and mute man, the Pharisees said, "The man drives out devils only through Beelzebul, the chief of the devils" (Mt 12:24). Then they demanded that Jesus work some miraculous signs to prove that he was God. But he refused, knowing that no extraordinary event could *prove* God's presence and love to "an evil and unfaithful generation" (Mt 12:39a).

When an observer of a miracle is morally disposed to see God's action, he is changed by the event. Some conversion occurs within him. The catch of fish changed Peter, James and John, who "left everything and followed [Jesus]" (Lk 5:11b). All four elements that could make an event miraculous came together and transformed their lives. The event meant much more to them than fish. They realized that God was calling them to a life of service.

The Meaning of Miracles

Miracles hold different meanings for different people. Those with a *non-incarnational approach* value them as their primary way to experience God. They believe that God dwells in his holy world, and we dwell in our godless, evil one. The sacred (heaven) and the profane (earth) do not mix. The non-incarnational idea of miracles holds that we cannot break out of our sinful world to touch God, but to show us that he cares, occasionally God miraculously breaks into our physical world in response to earnest prayer.

People with an *apologetic approach* to miracles value them as a way to *prove* religious truth. Apologists would say that Jesus' healings proved he was divine. Miracles sometimes do have this *effect* on people, but this says nothing about the *reason* they are done.[5] Jesus didn't do miracles to prove he was God; he did them to bring forth the kingdom of God. Some saw these miracles as having a divine meaning. They "believed." Others, such as the Pharisees, saw Jesus' miracles but never realized he was the Son of God. The same situation exists now. If the apologetic approach to miracles were valid, then every person today who experienced an extraordinary event would come to believe that Jesus is Lord.

The *incarnational, sacramental approach* to miracles values them as an integral part of the kingdom of God. It says that miracles are the good news in action. As discussed in Chapter 4, the good news in action means the kingdom of God already is truly present here on earth. Miracles are a direct, frontal attack on the kingdom of darkness, which also still remains here, but in a defeated form.[6]

As in Jesus' time, today's miracles say "this *is* the kingdom of God." Some are physically extraordinary events, such as a man's complete remission from terminal cancer. Others are emotional or spiritual events, such as a woman's healing of the emotional wounds of rape. Miracles aren't the *only* way to experience God, but these extraordinary events bring God into people's lives in a profound way, making his words come to life. Miracles say, "Look, I am making the whole of creation new" (Rv 21:5).

Miracles in Ministry

The way ministers view miracles profoundly influences their ministry.

Miracles as magic: Although they would vehemently deny it, some ministers use magical thinking in an attempt to *make* miracles happen. It's their job to *force* healing to happen through the use of magic powers. If the desired result does not occur instantly, they push harder. Like Lila (Chapter 2), they order people around and command them to do things (e.g., "Throw away your crutches!").

People using magical thinking want to enlist the help of powers that are favorable to their cause. They wish to be masters over their own earthly life and the lives of others. They do this by using any words or objects that will help their cause. The objects may be religious ones, even a crucifix. The words may be rites, prayers, or scripture verses. These details are unimportant, because the major concern with magical thinking is control.

When miracles are magic, emotions dominate ministry. The minister feels anxious because she feels responsible for producing results. She thinks she is accountable to God for people's healings. This creates a tension in the minister that infects her supplicants. Emotions rise to a fevered pitch. Ministers find promises in the Bible, fix their attention on them, and push them on their supplicants. ("It says in Luke 11:9 'Ask, and it will be given to you.' Lord, we *believe* that *right now* you're healing Molly's bursitis.") Sometimes devotions to saints are used in the same way, as a way to *make* something happen.

The magical approach to miracles may use religious terminology and actions without being religious. For instance, wearing a cross can be a witness to the world of one's Christian faith, or it can be a talisman to ward off bad luck. Interior disposition is what determines whether the action flows out of a religious or magical attitude.

The magical attitude focuses on controlling the forces of good and evil, even controlling God. On the other hand, the religious attitude sees oneself as dependent upon a loving, caring God who can be trusted. Human nature needs tangible, concrete signs such as rites, symbols, prayers, in order to experience God's presence. These signs enhance an awareness of being connected with God, but the religious attitude recognizes that they possess no innate power. For example, Jesus' name can be used as a profanity or as a powerful expression of faith.[7]

The lure of magic can be overwhelming for ministers of religious healing, but we can resist its attraction if we turn to Jesus and follow his example. In the desert, Satan tempted Jesus to use magic ("If you are Son of God, tell this stone to turn into a loaf" [Lk 4:3]). Jesus refused, both then and later ("Then save yourself if your are God's son and come down from the cross!" [Mt 27:40b]). Magic was contrary to his whole orientation, which was one of total dependence upon the Father.

Miracles as physical phenomena: Some people focus their entire ministry on miracles that involve just physical phenomena, such as a blind person regaining her sight. Their fixation implies that the transformation of someone's body is more important than the transformation of his mind and spirit. It ignores those scripture passages that show how Jesus' ministry brought God's redeeming action into the full spectrum of people's lives: physical, emotional, and spiritual. As "imitators of God" (Eph 5:1, *NIV*), we are called to do likewise.

When we open our eyes to the fullness of God's action in healing ministry, we realize that a supplicant's reconciliation with God can be as wondrous an event as the instant healing of, say, a broken ankle. Both point to the kingdom of God, but physical healing benefits people only for this life, whereas reconciliation with God lasts for eternity.

Ministers who see miracles only in the physical realm may forget that these phenomena do not *prove* anything. Physical anomalies can occur with no thought of the supernatural, e.g., some cancers go into spontaneous remission through no intervention by either science or ministry. They just cease. By themselves, these experiences don't prove the existence of God, the holiness of a minister or the faith of a supplicant.

Miracles as the only *way to experience God*:   Ministry that is built on this belief easily leads to frenzy because, here, God is present only in the supernatural and the spectacular, not in the natural and the ordinary. Therefore, the entire ministry revolves around miracles rather than around God.

When ministers believe that miracles are the only way to experience God, supplicants are vigorously urged to rouse their faith and "claim their healing." Later, supplicants may report the ministry felt like emotional abuse. Bystanders look on the scene like spectators at a circus. Peace flees, as does order and worship. With or without dramatic results, "miracle ministry" causes great harm to the ministry of religious healing.

Miracles as non-*physical events only*:   Some ministers of religious healing insist that transcendent physical events rarely, if ever, occur. They believe the kingdom of God takes place only in the ordinary and therefore fail to look and pray for the extraordinary. Here, someone asking for prayer for healing from multiple sclerosis will receive prayer for acceptance of the disease, not a cure from it. The ministers expect nothing to happen physically, and sure enough, it doesn't. People who see miracles only in non-physical events shortchange both the supplicant and God. The moment may have arrived when physical healing is possible, but it will pass if no one is open to recognizing it. Like the people in Jesus' home town of Nazareth (Mt 13:54–58), God cannot do many miracles if people lack expectant trust ("faith"). And those who lack expectant trust are as likely to be ministers as much as supplicants.

Miracles as a part of God's loving care: Ministers with an incarnational approach to healing believe that God is present in the ordinary *and* the extraordinary, the physical and the non-physical. Their both/and style of ministry allows them to see God's loving care in the subtle and the obvious, in the scientific and the religious, in the psychological and the spiritual.[8] They see miracles that others miss by failure of vision or failure of expectation. Faith enables them to discern the myriad ways God wants to usher in his kingdom in each situation.

When we adopt an incarnational approach to healing, we avoid the temptation to be obsessed with the spectacular. Instead, we can focus on God, leaving him in charge of results. A God-focus enables supplicants to continue on their spiritual journey, free from over-dependence on us. Best of all, as we keep our eyes on God instead of miracles, we come to realize the truth that something good *always* happens in good ministry. Our God of love constantly surprises us in astounding ways.

Conclusion

We began this book by saying that religious healing is a 2,000-year-old treasure in the Catholic church that has been pastorally ignored for several centuries. As a result, today's parishioners lack an experience of God meeting them in their various needs for healing, especially physical and emotional healing.

Changing the current situation will require great effort on everyone's part. First, church leaders must be willing to shoulder the added responsibility of finding ways to provide good, sound training and supervision of lay people. Secondly, prospective ministers of religious healing need to invest time, money and energy to become competent in a ministry that will give them no financial reward. Finally, parishes that already strain to meet their other responsibilities must make it a priority to respond to Jesus' commission to heal his hurting people.

Can this transformation occur? Can the ministry of religious healing find a home in normal parish life? We think so. It's already happening in some parts of the United States, and with God's grace, it can happen everywhere. For this to take place, however, we need to grasp the vision of what the Body of Christ can do for hurting people. We have been given the power that raised Jesus from the dead:

> I ask that your minds may be opened to see his light, so that you will know what is the hope to which he has called you, how rich are the wonderful blessings he promises his people, and how very great is his power at work in us who believe. This power in us is the same as the mighty strength which he used when he raised Christ from death, and seated him at his right side in the heavenly world (Eph 1:18–20, *TEV*).

Summary

An obsession with extraordinary physical events takes people's eyes off of God and puts them onto results and "healers." This discredits healing ministry.

The *popular view* of miracles sees them as events that defy the laws of nature. This divides the world into opposing parts and creates the belief that God is mostly absent from the natural world. This, in turn, leads to a style of ministry where the goal is to rouse God to come down to earth and "do" a miracle.

The popular view leads to a number of reactions, including: (1) acceptance of the situation; (2) ignoring the whole issue; (3) discounting the existence of miracles because they can't be proved by using empirical methods; (4) a belief that miracles existed in the early church but no longer do; (5) explaining away so-called "miracles" in scripture by saying the stories were a way to convey deep truths to an uneducated society.

The *expanded view* of miracles contains four elements: (1) transcendence — physical or otherwise; (2) a religious context; (3) sign value; and (4) a moral disposition in the observer.

Miracles hold different meanings for different people, depending on whether they view them (1) as magic; (2) as primarily physical phenomena; (3) as the *only* way to experience God; (4) as *non*-physical events only; or (5) as a part of God's loving care.

The way ministers view miracles affects their ministry:

(1)   Those who treat them as magic, as primarily physical phenomena or as the *only* way to experience God, adopt a style of ministry that revolves around miracles. It tends to be frenzied because it focuses on *results* instead of on God.

(2)   Those who believe that transcendent physical events never occur lack the faith to enable God to bring about those events. They short-change their supplicants.

(3)   Those with an incarnational approach focus their ministry on God and see miracles that surpass physical phenomena. They experience the truth that something good *always* happens in good ministry.

Endnotes

Chapter 1

1.   Throughout this book we frequently mention the problems created at large healing services. Often these problems are caused by badly trained and/or power-oriented superstars. Even at their best, however, large healing services lack two ingredients essential to pastoral ministry: personalized care and the opportunity for long-term follow-up ministry. Having said this, we acknowledge that a number of competent, holy ministers have weighed the built-in negatives of these services and have decided that the disadvantages are off-set by the healings that do occur. These healings can reveal God's love and presence to those who experience them and those who witness them.

2.   For a brief explanation on how the anointing of the sick came to be a sacrament for the dying, see Morton Kelsey's *Healing and Christianity* (San Francisco: Harper & Row, 1973, pp. 207–210).

3.   The church still has a ritual for the last rites, which is called *viaticum* (literally, "on the way with you"). The term applies to eucharist which is given to dying people for their journey to God. It's actual usage is rare because few who are on the verge of death are able to consume anything by mouth. The more common practice, then, is still to administer the sacrament of anointing of the sick and/or use prayers from the "Commendation of the Dying," which is contained in *Pastoral Care of the Sick*.

4.   McBrien, Richard P. *Catholicism.* San Francisco: Harper & Row, 1981, p. 785.

5.   *General Introduction, Pastoral Care of the Sick: Rites of Anointing and Viaticum.* New York: Catholic Book Publishing Co., 1983, Par. 5.

6.   The sacrament of anointing of the sick is intended for physical and emotional healing. The sacrament of reconciliation is intended for spiritual healing.

7.   In *Healing and Christianity* (p. 223), Kelsey writes, "By a strange quirk of logic it is permissible to remove medically the results of man's sins (sickness), but it is not quite correct to believe that God will do it himself if asked in prayer or invoked through sacraments."

8.   *General Introduction*, Par. 1, 4.

9.   Talley, Thomas. "Healing: Sacrament or Charism?" *Worship*: Vol. 46, No. 9 (November 1972), p. 518.

10.   In *Community, Church and Healing* (London: Darton, Longman & Todd, 1963, chapter 8), physician R. A. Lambourne notes the frequency of healing works in the gospels. Five different Greek words express these healings. Two of them

always describe medical healing, another means cleansing from leprosy, and another (rarely-used) means "restore whole." The fifth Greek word for curing/healing is *sozein*. Its Latin version is *salus*, from which English derives both salvation and salve.

In scripture, when *sozein* refers to a medical situation, it is translated as *healed* or *made whole*. When used in a theological setting, it usually is translated as *saved*. *Sozein* is the word for curing/healing seen most often in the New Testament. If health means only physical wellness, why didn't the gospel writers use a word that means only medical healing? The writers deliberately chose an inclusive word because healing and salvation were so intertwined in Hebrew tradition and in the early church that they were nearly indistinguishable. "Salvation" meant health of body, mind *and* soul. We need to return to this truth and to remember that the churh exists to bring us into health, into *sozein* in all its meanings.

11. *Living Worship*: Vol. 8, No. 7 (September 1972), a publication of the Liturgical Conference.

12. *General Introduction*, Par. 43.

Chapter 2

1. Theologian Richard P. McBrien discusses interpretations of the word "body" in *The Church in the Thought of Bishop John Robinson* (Philadelphia: Westminster Press, 1966, cf. p. 33).

2. This statement in no way diminishes the fact that God calls us into a one-on-one personal relationship with him. A relationship with Jesus is the most intimate one possible between two persons, one of whom is divine.

3. Haughey, John C. *The Conspiracy of God: The Holy Spirit in Men*. Garden City, NY: Doubleday, 1973, p. 94.

4. Paul uses "in Christ" to describe our being a part of the Body of Christ. When done "in Christ," our acts are truly Christ's acts, and his acts are truly ours because we form one person, the total Christ.

We are not "in Christ" as a fish is in water. Instead, we are more like a drop of water in a river. The river is the entirety. Without each individual drop, the river would not exist! The weakness of this analogy is that a drop of water loses its individuality by being in the river's entirety, but the Christian does not lose his identity by being "in Christ."

For further discussion of this subject, see: Fernand Prat, S.J., *The Theology of Saint Paul, Vol. II* (Westminster, MD: The Newman Book Store, 1952, p. 298).

5. Two health care professionals who come to mind are Dr. Bernie Siegel, author of *Peace, Love and Healing* (New York: Harper & Row, 1989), and Dr. Carl Simonton, co-author of *Getting Well Again* (New York: Bantam, 1978).

6. Vatican II recognized the need for shared responsibility of lay and clergy alike to serve God as members of the Body of Christ. Since then, church leaders

have been striving to heighten sound, effective lay involvement. Richard McBrien addresses this subject in *Ministry: A Theological, Pastoral Handbook* (San Francisco: Harper & Row, 1987, cf. pp. 114–115). Jesuit theologian Donald L. Gelpi asserts that lay people "have the right to expect that the Christian community provide them with the means of deepening and developing their gift of service." See *God Breathes the Spirit in the World* (Wilmington, DE: Michael Glazier, 1988, p. 76).

Chapter 3

1. Why should ministers of religious healing care about what health is? At first glance, the question seems to belong in a dictionary or a doctoral thesis. But knowing the *religious* meaning of health will shed light on why the ministry of religious healing exists. Without this understanding, pastoral care to the sick goes awry. Those who grasp the religious meaning of health are able to keep their eyes fixed on the goal of healing ministry.

2. Fritjof Capra describes this body-as-machine model in his book *The Turning Point: Science, Society and the Rising Culture* (New York: Bantam Books, 1982, p. 123).

3. Eric J. Cassell. *The Healer's Art: A New Approach to the Doctor-Patient Relationship*. Philadelphia: Lippincott, 1976, p. 48.

4. Bernie S. Siegel, M.D. *Peace, Love, and Healing*. New York: Harper & Row, 1989, p. 121 (emphasis added).

5. *Ibid.*, p. 16.

6. *Ibid.*, p. 20. Webster's dictionary defines a placebo as "a harmless, unmedicated preparation given as a medicine to a patient merely to humor him, or used as a control in testing the efficacy of another, medicated substance."

This popular interpretation of a placebo's being fake as a way of humoring a patient puts the doctor in the role of a trickster and the patient in the role of a fool. The medical community now is beginning to see placebos in a different light, thanks to the efforts of respected physicians and researchers like Howard Brody (*Placebos and the Philosophy of Medicine*, Chicago: University of Chicago Press, 1980) and Michael Jospe (*The Placebo Effect in Healing*, Lexington: Heath and Co., 1978).

On p. 21 of *Peace, Love, and Healing*, Dr. Siegel writes: "In an essay entitled 'The Mysterious Placebo,' Norman Cousins gets to the heart of how it's done. . . .: 'The placebo is an emissary between the will to live and the body. But the emissary is expendable. If we can liberate ourselves from tangibles, we can connect hope and the will to live directly to the ability of the body to meet great threats and challenges.' What the placebo suggests to us is that we may be able to change what takes place in our bodies by changing our state of mind."

7. *Ibid.*, p. 36.

8.   Kohlenberg, Robert J., Ph.D. *Migraine Relief: A Personal Treatment Program.* New York: Harper & Row, 1983.

9.   *Ibid.*, pp. 51, 52.

10.   "That divine power of his has freely bestowed on us everything necessary for a life of genuine piety, through knowledge of him who called us by his own glory and power. By virtue of them he has bestowed on us the great and precious things he promised, so that through these you who have fled a world corrupted by lust might become *sharers of the divine nature*" (2 Pt 1:3–4, *NAB*).

11.   In *Models of the Church* (Garden City, NY: Doubleday, 1974, pp. 49–50), Jesuit Avery Dulles explains our transformation: "... What is new in the New Covenant [is] that men [and women] are brought into a consciously affirmed filial relationship to God. We become by adoption what Jesus Christ is by origin: sons [and daughters] of God."

12.   Mooth, Verla A. *Forgiveness and Healing.* Pecos, NM: Dove Publications, leaflet #39.

13.   Dulles, p. 60.

14.   In *Catholicism* (San Francisco: Harper & Row, 1981) Richard P. McBrien explains this theology: "The Catholic tradition has always been insistent that the grace of God is given to us...as a gift that elevates us to a new and unmerited level of existence.... By the grace of Christ we enter into a new relationship of communion with God, and we are transformed interiorly by the Spirit of Christ.... We are, in fact, called to a participation in the life of God through Jesus Christ" (pp. 151–52).

15.   Willard, Dallas. *The Spirit of the Disciplines: Understanding How God Changes Lives.* San Francisco: Harper & Row, 1988, pp. 35–36.

16.   Haughey, John C. *The Conspiracy of God: The Holy Spirit in Men.* Garden City, NY: Doubleday, 1973, pp. 92–93.

17.   Brown, Raymond. *The Gospel According to John*, Vol. 2, The Anchor Bible, Vol. 29. Garden City, NY: Doubleday, 1966, p. 506.

Chapter 4

1.   O'Meara, Thomas Franklin, O.P. *Theology of Ministry.* New York/Mahwah: Paulist Press, 1983, p. 4.

2.   McBrien, Richard P. *Ministry: A Theological, Pastoral Handbook.* San Francisco: Harper & Row, 1987, p. 15.

3.   O'Meara, pp. 26, 29.

4.   Shea, John. "Is the Pain Worth the Gain? What it Means to Take up Your Cross." *U. S. Catholic*: March 1990, p. 9.

5. Bernardin, Joseph Cardinal. *In Service of One Another: Pastoral Letter on Ministry*. Chicago: The Chicago Catholic Publishing Co., 1985.

Chapter 5

1. M. Scott Peck, M.D. *The Road Less Traveled*. New York: Simon & Schuster, 1978, p. 120.

2. For a better understanding of the church's view of itself as a "perfect society," see Avery Dulles, S.J., *Models of the Church* (Garden City, NY: Doubelday, 1974, chapter 2).

3. Throughout the entire history of the church, theologians have struggled with how best to explain its sinfulness. Some models of the church are better than others in understanding this issue. See chapter 3 of *Models of the Church*, especially pp. 50–51 for a discussion of this problem.

4. Chapters 2 and 3 of Leo's book, *Healing Ministry: A Practical Guide* (Kansas City, MO: Sheed & Ward, 1994) explore the dynamics of team ministry in more depth.

5. An interview with Parker Palmer, "Getting Out Would Do Your Faith a World of Good." *U.S. Catholic*: February 1991, p. 11.

6. A good resource for exploring the psychology of expectations can be found in Jerome D. Frank's book *Persuasion and Healing* (New York: Schocken Books, 1974, chapter 5).

7. The gift of knowledge is one of the authentic gifts of the Spirit described in 1 Cor 12:4–11. But its use in large healing services can wreak havoc. Say a leader discerns—accurately—that at that moment God intends to heal someone's breast cancer. Three women in the room know they have this disease. The one to whom this knowledge is directed feels too demoralized to believe God is speaking to her. Without a minister to personally help her grow in faith, she leaves the service unhealed. But one of the other sufferers grasps onto the leader's message like a drowning person. Thrilled, she announces the good news to her doctor, but then discovers she still has cancer. The common response in this scenario is to feel devastated with despair and false guilt. To maximize its power and avoid the above problem, the gift of knowledge should be used in a *personal* way, prayerfully addressed to a specific person who knows the Lord is speaking directly to her.

Chapter 6

1. Officials of the church are rightfully concerned that no impression be given that a lay person is administering the sacrament of anointing of the sick. The oil the prayer minister used was blessed by a *priest* for *lay* use; it was not the oil blessed by a *bishop* for the sacrament, which Leo used in anointing Anthony. When lay ministers use blessed oil in ministering religious healing they must make it clear that they are not administering a sacrament. Various formularies for blessing oil for

lay use are available, e.g., *A Book of Blessings* (Ottawa: Canadian Conference of Catholic Bishops, 1981, p. 361).

2.   It may seem strange to think of worshipers coming before the Lord with a need. Although sometimes we are conscious of our needs in worship, frequently we are not. We may come to worship out of habit or in an unreflective manner. Nevertheless, when we come before God, we always come in need. There is no other way: we are totally dependent on God. We have nothing to give him except what he first has given to us. The need may be very general, e.g., a need to hear God's word or to experience his love, or it may be specific, e.g., a need for forgiveness or healing.

3.   For more about healing ministry as worship, see chapter 1 of Leo's book *Healing Ministry: A Practical Guide* (Kansas City, MO: Sheed & Ward, 1994)

4.   We recommend Fran Ferder's *Words Made Flesh* (Notre Dame: Ave Maria Press, 1988), Thomas Hart's *The Art of Christian Listening* (New York/Mahwah: Paulist Press, 1980), and section 2 of *The Healing Team.*

5.   Chapter 14 of *Healing Ministry: A Practical Guide* goes into more depth on prayer of affirmation.

6.   Prayers of petition focus on one's own, personal needs. Prayers of intercession focus on the needs of others — in this chapter, the supplicant.

7.   This is a vast simplification of a challenging theology. Jesuit John H. Wright discusses it in his book *A Theology of Christian Prayer* (New York: Pueblo Publishing, 1979, pp. 67–81). When we intercede as the Body of Christ, we bring with us all of creation that has been reconciled to the Father by Christ. In the context of worship, intercession unites us completely with God's loving purpose for a particular supplicant *and* for the whole of creation. The union is so complete that redeemed creation becomes an instrument for God's loving power to set things right. This creation includes surgery, doctors, loved ones, counselors, medication and therapy as well as such spiritual supports as prayer ministers and sacraments.

8.   This may be a shocking statement unless we reflect upon our own experience of its truth. Consider the difference between our response to a power outage at home versus at an unfamiliar place. At home, we "know" (i.e., have an image of) the path between a flashlight and us. Using this image, we reach our goal with a minimum of panic or bruised shins. In a strange place, however, we glue ourselves to the spot where we stood when the power went out. No mental images exist, so purposeful action is impossible.

What holds true for physical surroundings also holds true for our sense of self. Through play, imitation, and contact with others, children develop an image of themselves that determines their careers, their choices of relationships, and their basic view of life. Without *some* self-image — positive or negative — they cannot act.

Much harm occurs as a result of warped or absent images. People fail to make good choices when their view of themselves and others is distorted. If they cannot accurately see their giftedness and the world's opportunities, they stumble through life making poor or hurtful choices. An intelligent child with a learning disability images herself as stupid — then acts accordingly — because classmates and teachers *tell* her she's stupid. A sexually abused child feels "dirty" and "bad" because that's the message his abuser gave him.

Distorted or absent images create pain that ministers of religious healing can help ease. No image is cast in concrete. It *can* change through various means. One of those means is the use of praying with imagery. The following are excellent resources for learning more about the use of imagery in the church's healing ministry:

Droege, Thomas A. *The Faith Factor in Healing*. Philadelphia: Trinity Press International, 1991.

Jackson, Edgar N. *The Role of Faith in the Process of Healing*. Minneapolis: Winston Press, 1981.

Scientific knowledge about mental imagery fits into a new field of medicine called psychoneuroimmunology. The specialty is investigating the mind/body connection in helpful ways, but some investigators have been influenced by the philosophy and spiritual practices of Eastern religions and New Age thought. Therefore Christians need to exercise discretion in using their recommended practices in prayer ministry. (Droege covers this subject in his above-mentioned book.)

Bearing in mind this caution, the following non-Christian books contain useful information about imagery:

Benson, Herbert. *The Mind/Body Effect*. New York: Berkley Books, 1979.

Bry, Adelaide. *Visualization: Directing the Movies of Your Mind*. New York: Barnes & Noble, 1978.

9.   Using scripture to pray with images is a Jesuit tradition that St. Ignatius Loyola described in his *Spiritual Exercises*, a guidebook for self-discipline and prayer.

10.   Several physicians write about the effectiveness of imagery in healing physical illnesses, including Bernie Siegel in *Peace, Love, and Healing* (New York: Harper & Row, 1989), and Carl Simonton, et al., in *Getting Well Again* (New York: Bantam, 1980). The latter book is especially useful in dealing with cancer, although we do not recommend chapter 15 ("Finding Your Inner Guide to Health") because we believe that an "inner guide" that is cut off from God can deceive people with false messages from themselves or from spirits other that the Holy Spirit.

Chapter 7

1.   An excellent book that gives detailed information on the practice of various disciplines necessary for an ordered Christian life is Dallas Willard's *The Spirit of the Disciplines: Understanding How God Changes Lives* (San Francisco: Harper & Row, 1988). For prayer, see especially pp. 185–188.

2.   In pp. 33-49 *Healing Ministry: A Practical Guide*, Leo describes the process of the cycle of ministry. The cycle involves, first, assessing the situation, then determining a plan for ministry, then implementing the plan, and finally evaluating the results. This brings the ministry full circle back to assessing the situation.

Part of this cycle takes place during preparation for ministry. Before each session with a supplicant, teams need to take 15–30 minutes to pray together, anoint one another, and establish a *tentative* plan of action for the session. Taking time to debrief after a supplicant leaves is also critically important for the success of healing ministry.

3.   Tugwell, Simon, O.P. *Did You Receive the Spirit?* New York: Paulist Press, 1972, pp. 79–80.

4.   St. Thomas, ST 2a2ae, 129.3 ad 4, as quoted in *The Catholic Encyclopedia*, 1967 edition.

5.   O'Meara, p. 170.

Chapter 8

1.   A surprising number of people keep a journal, especially during times of stress or change. Supplicants sometimes share selected entries with their prayer team and report that both the journaling and the sharing of their writings are sources of healing for them.

2.   Frank, Jerome. *Persuasion and Healing*. New York: Schocken Books, 1973, p. 330.

3.   *Ibid.*, p. 72.

4.   As footnoted in Chapter 7, Dorothy's prayer team used the cycle of ministry with her (assessing the situation, determining a plan of action for ministry, implementing the plan, then evaluating the results). Often a team goes through several cycles of ministry before it is possible to assess the basic need. After two cycles of ministry, Dorothy's team realized that her basic need was for spiritual healing in the aftermath of an abortion. Then they were able to devise a plan for ministry and implement it.

5.   "Project Rachel" is an international Christian ministry of post-abortion reconciliation. Many Catholic dioceses in the United States have trained priests who have been specially authorized by their bishop to engage in this ministry. To access the names of Rachel priests within a given diocese, ministers can phone their diocesan office *or* The National Office of Post-Abortion Reconciliation and Healing at (800) 5WE-CARE.

Chapter 9

1.   Frank, Jerome. *Persuasion and Healing*. New York: Schocken Books, 1973, p. 314.

2.   Frank, Jerome. "The Role of Hope in Psychotherapy." *International Journal of Psychiatry*: Vol. 5 (1968), pp. 383–95.

3. Richter, C. P. "On the Phenomenon of Sudden Death in Animals and Man." *Psychosomatic Medicine*: Vol. 19 (1957), pp. 191–98. Richter reports an experiment that helps us understand unexplained, sudden deaths in both humans and animals, such as death brought on by a curse. In his experiment, wild rats were placed in a stressful situation from which they could not escape by either fight or flight. They were restrained, then placed in a tank of water, where they had to swim continuously. The rats quit swimming in a matter of minutes, long before the depletion of their normal endurance, which could last as long as 80 hours.

If the rats were briefly released several times from the stressful situation and then reimmersed in the water, the rapid "giving up" disappeared. They swam hour after hour. Richter concluded that the brief respite from the "impossible-to-escape" situation convinced the rats that escape was possible. Temporary relief allowed the animals to "imagine a tolerable future."

4. Frank, Jerome. "The Role of Hope in Psychotherapy." p. 383ff.

5. Pruyser, Paul. "The Phenomenology and Dynamics of Hoping." *The Journal of the Scientific Study of Religion*: Vol. 3 (1963), pp. 93–94.

6. Lynch, W. F. *Images of Hope: Imagination as Healer of the Hopeless*. New York: New American Library, 1965.

7. Styron, William. *Darkness Visible: A Memoir of Madness*. New York: Random House, 1990, p. 76.

8. Weatherhead, Leslie D. *Psychology, Religion and Healing*. New York: Abingdon-Cokesbury, 1951, pp. 423–435.

9. *Ibid.*, pp. 430, 432.

10. *Ibid.*, p. 26, emphasis added.

11. *Ibid.*, p. 425.

Chapter 10

1. Weatherhead, Leslie D. *Psychology, Religion and Healing*. New York: Abingdon-Cokesbury, 1951, p. 425.

2. In those instances when a person's life is in danger, it's necessary to take temporary control of the situation if the person is unwilling to cooperate. Since Dorothy was considering suicide, she needed immediate help. Because she was willing to go to a psychiatrist, her husband did not need to take control of her free will. Prayer ministry, however, was an option Dorothy could accept or reject.

3. For more on the subject of sacramentals, see Robert L. Kinast's *Sacramental Pastoral Care: Integrating Resources for Ministry* (New York: Pueblo, 1988).

4. What we object to in the phrase "offering up one's suffering" is the belief that God somehow "gets" something out of our suffering. This puts God in the

role of a monstrous, sadistic being, which is blasphemy. But there is an acceptable meaning to this phrase that needs to be recognized and respected.

Even if a sick person isn't cured, the Body of Christ can help him gain a victory. Graced by God, the sufferer can refuse to be demoralized by disease or to be alienated from God and the Christian community. He can maintain hope that God can bring good out of evil. In this way, sickness can be converted into a condition that can be lived positively as a Christian. It is a partial sharing in the victory of Christ over the power of evil, which strives to kill the *spirit* as well as the *body*. What is being "offered up," then, is not the suffering of being sick, but rather the refusal to be mastered by that suffering. God rejoices, not in the sick person's pain, but in his refusal to relinquish faith and hope in God's goodness even in the midst of pain. This, as article #3 in the instruction to the rite of the pastoral care of the sick says, can be a valuable witness to the whole church. It demonstrates the power of God's grace to triumph over evil.

Chapter 11

1.   See Colin Brown's *Miracles and the Critical Mind* (Grand Rapids: Eerdmans, 1984) for a thorough discussion of the history of the various responses to the question of miracles.

2.   See "Theology of Miracles," *New Catholic Encyclopedia* (New York: McGraw-Hill, 1967, Vol. IX, p. 890b).

3.   See, for example, Robert W. Gleason, "Miracles and Contemporary Theology," *Thought*. Vol. 37, No. 144 (Spring 1962), pp. 12–34. Also M. A. H. Melinsky, *Healing Miracles: An Examination*. . . , (London: Mowbray & Co., 1968).

4.   See "Moral Miracle," *New Catholic Encyclopedia*, New York: McGraw-Hill, 1967, Vol. IX, pp. 884a and 891a.

5.   See David Stanley, "Salvation and Healing," *The Way*: Vol. 10 (1970), pp. 298–317.

6.   See James Kallas, *Jesus and the Power of Satan* (Philadelphia: Westminster Press, 1968, p. 155).

7.   For more on this subject, see Lawrence F. X. Brett's *Redeemed Creation: Sacraments Today* (Wilmington, DE: M. Glazier, 1984).

8.   For more on the incarnational view of the world, see William Barclay's *The Mind of St. Paul* (New York: HarperCollins, 1986, pp. 32–41).